What's in Our Food

What's in Our Food

*Fact and Fiction about Fat and Fiber,
Vitamins and Minerals,
Nutrients and Contaminants*

Mia Parsonnet, M.D.

Illustrations by Kathy Cadow Parsonnet

MADISON BOOKS

LANHAM • NEW YORK • LONDON

Published by Madison Books
4720 Boston Way
Lanham, Maryland 20706

3 Henrietta Street
London WC2E 8LU, England

Library of Congress Cataloging-in-Publication Data

Parsonnet, Mia.
What's in our food: fact and fiction about fat and fiber, vitamins and minerals,
nutrients and contaminants / Mia Parsonnet; illustrations by Kathy Cadow Parsonnet.
p. cm.
Includes index.
1. Food—Composition. 2. Food—Analysis. I. Title.
TX531.P28   1996   95-51724 613.2—dc20 CIP

ISBN 1-56833-049-9 (pbk. : alk. paper)

Distributed by National Book Network

⊖™ The paper used in this publication meets the minimum requirements of
American National Standard for Information Sciences—Permanence of
Paper for Printed Library Materials, ANSI Z39.48–1984.
Manufactured in the United States of America.

Contents

Chapter 7

Chapter 8

Chapter 9

Tables and Charts

Acknowledgment

I want to thank the two busiest people I know for their immeasurable help: my husband, Dr. Victor Parsonnet, for his patience and unstinting support at every step of this undertaking, and my daughter, Dr. Julie Parsonnet, for her diligent and savvy critique of the manuscript.

M.P.

Introduction

We are constantly bombarded by ads that tell us what is good for us and what we shouldn't do without. But which of these claims is true, and which is double-talk? What do we really need in our daily diet, and how do we get it?

Many of us know more about the mix we feed our African violets and the gasoline we put in our cars than about the food we eat. We look at phosphorus and nitrogen in plant food, and at octanes and additives in gas, and hope that this attention will keep the flowers blooming and the engines humming. When it comes to ourselves, however, we tend to be less well-informed, perhaps in the mistaken belief that the body will take care of itself.

Our ideas about nutrition are changing constantly. There are no guarantees that what we know today will not be discredited tomorrow or, on the other hand, that some far-out claims won't ultimately prove their worth. Still, the field of nutrition has a solid base, enhanced in recent years by a huge amount of interest and study.

This book is intended to provide basic information to the consumer about all the substances we eat. I have made an effort to present as fact what is fact, to identify conjectures and fads, and to demystify some terms and concepts that have become part of our vocabulary, whether we quite understand them or not.

CHAPTER 1

Protein: The Stuff of Life

The uniqueness of living things is linked primarily to proteins. They are components of every cell and tissue, and comprise at least half of the dry weight of animals.

Protein molecules are large and complex. They consist of long chains of **amino acids,** the protein "building blocks." After a protein meal the body splits these large molecules into the constituent amino acids and fashions them to form *new* proteins, characteristic of the species and of the function they are to serve.

Adequate protein intake is essential for growth and cell regeneration. Young children require a minimum of an ounce of pure protein daily. For nonpregnant adults the amount is about 2 ounces. This sounds like very little, but foods do not consist of *pure* protein. It takes about 3 or 4 ounces of meat or fish, or a quart of milk, or 5 eggs to provide just one ounce (28 gm) of protein. The same amount, though not the same quality of protein can also be obtained from 4 cups of cooked spaghetti or 2½ cups of cooked lima beans. The advantage of *animal* proteins is that they are more concentrated and contain a greater assortment of desirable amino acids. The advantage of *vegetable* proteins is that they are much less likely to be linked to fat.

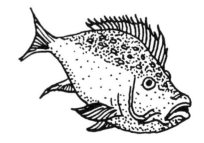

The healthy body tries to pre-

1

serve protein; protein is utilized for fuel only when carbohydrate and fat stores have been depleted. Proteins and fats can be made into carbohydrates and be used for energy; proteins and carbohydrates can be converted to fat and be deposited as such, but neither fats nor carbohydrates can create proteins.

AMINO ACIDS

The characteristics and nutritional value of a protein are determined by the arrangement and type of its constituent amino acids. In human beings, about two dozen amino acids are necessary for good nutrition. Nine of them are called "essential." This does not mean that they contribute more to nutrition than nonessential ones; it simply means that they must be taken in the diet because the human body is unable to manufacture them from more basic food stuffs or from other amino acids.

The essential amino acids are histidine, isoleucine, leucine, lysine, methionine, (cystine can substitute in part), phenylalanine (tyrosine can substitute in part), threonine, tryptophan, and valine. Arginine is sometimes included in this list. It *can* be synthesized, but not always in sufficient amounts during maximum growth periods or at times of unusual bodily stress. The actual quantities needed of each amino acid are quite small.

For maximum nutritional benefit, a proper assortment of amino acids must be available *at the same time*. Animal proteins such as those found in meat, fish, eggs, and dairy products are more varied than vegetable proteins. Nevertheless, by being informed and selecting proper *combinations* of vegetable products, vegetarians can achieve good protein nutrition. Rice and red beans or rice and lentils, for example, are good sources as are chickpeas and sesame seeds or beans and cheese. All of these combinations are common in different parts of the world, and represent sound folk wisdom. The greatest potential hazard for strict vegetarians is a deficiency of Vitamin B_{12} and even that occurs only after years of abstinence from all animal products.

Except on very restricted diets (eating only one or two foods), deficiency of a single amino acid does not occur nor does general amino acid deficiency. Supplements are not recommended; they are expensive and may actually upset the desirable amino acid balance. Amino acid supplements have been touted to athletes as muscle builders. The best that can be said for them in this regard is that they are probably less harmful than anabolic steroids. Long-term effects of large doses are not yet known.

Two amino acids have received some special attention in recent years: tryptophan is reputed to have a calming effect because it is a precursor of serotonin; and tyrosine is said to act as a stimulant, increasing alertness and memory because it is a precursor of adrenaline. The efficacy of tryptophan has not been verified, and serious side effects have been reported (possibly due to a contaminant). Tyrosine is being tested in patients who suffer attacks of irresistible sleep (narcolepsy), but there is no evidence that it acts as an energizer in healthy people.

PURINES

In the body, purines are normal breakdown products of certain proteins. In some medical conditions, particularly in gout, purine metabolism is disturbed, and one of the purines, uric acid, rises in the blood and is deposited in the joints causing painful attacks of arthritis. In gout and several other diseases, foods with a high purine yield should be avoided.

Foods Highest in Purines
Organ meats: sweetbreads, liver, kidneys, brains
Seafood: anchovies, sardines, herring, scallops

Foods Lowest In Purines
Fruits and nuts
Dairy products
Eggs
Refined cereals and breads

FASCINATING FACTS ABOUT PROTEINS

- Brown eggs have the same nutritional value as white eggs.
- Red meat from free-grazing animals is leaner and tougher than the meat of domestic animals. It may also be healthier because it has a

more favorable ratio of different saturated fatty acids. That means that venison, buffalo, and goat meat are less likely to raise blood cholesterol than ranch-raised beef.

- The ancient Chinese began the cultivation of soybeans, a fine source of vegetable protein. Today the United States grows more soybeans than any other country in the world.
- Surplus protein in the diet is burned for energy or stored as fat. It does not add to muscle tissue or increase muscle power. The way to enlarge and strengthen muscles is to exercise them.
- A high-protein diet usually includes a lot of fat. In fact, some high-protein foods (like a fine steak) get more calories from fat than from protein. In a so-called healthy breakfast of orange juice, bacon and eggs, buttered toast, and a glass of milk, fat provides about 53 percent of the calories compared to only 15 percent of protein and 32 percent carbohydrate.

CHAPTER 2

Carbohydrates:
Complex and Otherwise

Carbohydrates are the most abundant source of food energy, and, for most people, provide the largest part of the diet. Ideally they should constitute about 55 percent of the caloric intake, with proteins supplying 15 percent and fats 30 percent. There are three basic carbohydrate groups: sugars or "simple carbohydrates," starches or "complex carbohydrates," and cellulose (fiber).

The best known *sugars* are sucrose (cane or beet sugar), fructose (fruit sugar), and lactose (milk sugar), but there are several others. Starches are derived chiefly from cereal grains; most vegetables and fruits *also* contain starches. The third group, *cellulose,* is not digested by humans; it is the fibrous part of most plant foods we eat, and provides useful roughage (and no calories).

Carbohydrates are more rapidly utilized than fats or proteins, and thus supply the quickest energy; this is particularly true of sugars, which tend to provide a fast but short-lived boost. Ultimately, most absorbed carbohydrates are broken down into the simplest of the sugars, glucose. This is the molecule that is carried in the blood stream for use by the various organs and tissues, there to be burned for energy, or to undergo another transformation that makes it suitable for storage.

Even the most restricted diet should include carbohydrates because, aside from their own intrinsic nutritional value, they also aid in the orderly utilization of protein and fat.

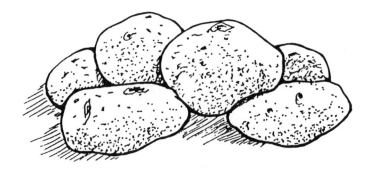

SUGAR AND OTHER CALORIC SWEETENERS

Honey bees were kept by the Egyptians more than 4,500 years ago. Sugar cane was described more than 2,000 years ago. It seems that man has always had a sweet tooth! In the United States we eat an average of 43 pounds of sugar a year.

Sugar provides calories (food energy) but offers virtually nothing in the way of vitamins or minerals. Since about a quarter of our daily calories are supplied by ordinary sugar (most of it in processed food), the rest of our diet had better be nutritious! In spite of its bad reputation sugar does *not* cause criminal behavior, hyperactivity, or diabetes (even though diabetes is a disease in which the blood sugar level may be high).

Table sugar provides 4 calories per gram, or 113 calories per ounce. It has less than half the calories of an equal weight of fat.

Sucrose is the most common variety and serves as our table sugar. It is obtained from sugar cane or sugar beets, and is marketed in granulated, powdered, or cube form. Sucrose is a disaccharide or double sugar, a composite of two simple sugars, glucose and fructose. In the course of digestion, sucrose is broken down into these two components.

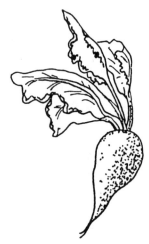

Invert sugar also consists of glucose and fructose, but is obtained by a chemical process that splits sucrose. It is marketed in liquid form, and is used chiefly in commercial food production.

Glucose is the main form of sugar normally carried in the blood stream. It supplies fuel to cells and tissues. The same formula is produced commercially from corn starch, and is known as corn sugar or **dextrose.**

Corn syrup is produced from cornstarch. It consists of glucose and fructose in varying proportions. The use of sweeteners derived from corn (corn syrup, corn sugar, dextrose) has increased tremendously over the last few decades.

Fructose, or fruit sugar, is found in honey and in sweet fruits. It is the sweetest of sugars, providing 1½ times as much sweetness as table sugar. The commercial form is known as **levulose.** Fructose is absorbed somewhat more slowly than sucrose and thus is less likely to produce sugar "highs and lows." It has no other nutritional advantage.

Honey consists of several sugars, chiefly fructose and glucose, in varying proportions. Because of its high fructose content, it achieves a specific degree of sweetness with somewhat fewer calories than table sugar. Tablespoon for tablespoon, however, it has more calories. Contrary to popular opinion, honey contains only trace amounts of vitamins and minerals. The color and flavor of various brands depend on the flowers on which the bees were feeding.

Raw sugar is sucrose obtained by direct evaporation of sugar cane juice. Unless dirt and other undesirable matter are removed, it is not recommended for human consumption.

Molasses is the residue after the extraction of sugar crystals from the raw sugar plant juice. It is the only sweetener that contains any significant amounts of vitamins (B_6 and other Bs) and minerals (iron, potassium, calcium).

Brown sugar is sucrose (table sugar) colored with varying amounts of caramel. It has no health advantage over white sugar. An exception is "Sugar in the Raw," a brand of light brown sugar which contains 15 percent molasses. (Unlike ordinary *raw* sugar, this product is clean.)

Lactose, or milk sugar, is found in the milk of mammals and is composed of glucose and galactose. It is made commercially from whey (the watery part of milk), and is used in the manufacture of drugs.

Galactose, also known as "brain sugar," is a component of the lactose in milk.

Maltose, or malt sugar, is composed of two glucose molecules. It is formed by fermentation or by chemical means. Maltose is used commercially in foods and drugs.

Maple syrup is primarily sucrose. When the liquid of the sap is boiled off, **maple sugar** is produced.

Sorbitol and **mannitol** (technically sugar alcohols) are found in some plants, but are also produced commercially from dextrose to be used, for example, in the manufacture of chewing gum and drug coatings. These sweeteners are about half as sweet as table sugar. Because sugar alcohols are metabolized differently from other sugars, they are preferred in food processed for diabetics.

Xylitol (wood sugar), another sugar alcohol, is made from birch wood, but is also found naturally in some fruits and berries. It is approximately as sweet as table sugar and is used like the other sugar alcohols. The safety of xylitol is under investigation.

NONCALORIC SWEETENERS

Since the introduction of diet soft drinks, artificial sweeteners have come into wider and wider use over the past 35 or 40 years. They are the sweeteners of choice for millions of people, and are used by manufacturers in many foods, beverages, and drugs. The vast majority of consumers use them for purposes of weight control, although there is in fact no documented evidence that this practice contributes to weight loss in the long run. (Americans have gotten fatter and fatter over the past years.)

Saccharin was discovered in 1879, and proved useful during sugar shortages in World Wars I and ll. In recent years several animal studies have cast doubt on the safety of saccharin, specifically when very large amounts were taken. For a time the product was removed from marketed foods and drinks, but it is now available once again and is used quite widely. *Sweet'n Low* and *Sugar Twin* are brands that contain saccharin. A liquid form, *Sugar Twin Plus,* contains both saccharine and aspartame.

Saccharine is 300 times sweeter than an equal weight of sugar. It has no calories.

Cyclamate, discovered about half a century ago, came into wide use in the 1950s and 1960s. In recent years its safety has come under scrutiny, and its use has been suspended. It may, however, be permitted again in the future.

Cyclamate is 30 times sweeter than sugar and has no calories. It is heat stable and dissolves easily in liquid.

Aspartame too has been subjected to a great deal of debate and much testing since it was discovered in 1965. For the last several years it has been approved for use in foods, beverages, and drugs. Except in individuals with a rare genetic disease (phenylketonuria or PKU), it is considered safe when taken in reasonable amounts.

Weight for weight aspartame actually has the same number of calories as sugar but it is 200 times as sweet and therefore only tiny amounts are needed. It does not retain this sweetness with prolonged heating, or when in solution for any length of time. The trade name is *NutraSweet.* It is used in *Equal.*

Acesulfame K is the newest approved artificial sweetener; *Sunette* is the trade name. It has no calories, is as sweet as aspartame, and is said to retain its qualities with heating and with prolonged storage. It is sold as *Sweet One.*

Several more artificial sweeteners are in the testing stage, among them **Sucralose,** a noncaloric relative of table sugar and 600 times sweeter, and **Alitame,** composed of amino acids and 2,000 times as sweet as sugar.

We may never be entirely certain that any artificial sweetener is totally safe. For the time being, none of them should be used by children and pregnant women. However, artificial sweeteners are now found in so many foods and beverages that they are hard to avoid.

FIBER

Dietary fiber, also called "roughage" or "bulk," consists of plant material that is indigestible and has no calories. Fiber does, however, affect digestion by drawing water into the stool, softening it and giving it more volume, and by regulating transit time through the intestinal tract. Fiber can also elicit the secretion of intestinal hormones and enzymes, and influence the absorption of nutrients; in that sense it may affect nutrition. Because it has a satiating effect, some dieters find high-fiber foods to be helpful in curbing hunger.

In recent years fiber has been categorized according to solubility in water. **Insoluble fiber,** mainly cellulose, exerts its action in the *lower* intestine, providing bulk. **Soluble fiber** acts on the *upper* intestine as well. There it affects the absorption of food stuffs. It may also have a cholesterol lowering effect, perhaps by altering bile acid metabolism. Current labeling laws permit no such direct claim, but allow a statement that relates high soluble fiber intake to a reduced risk of coronary heart disease.

As an aside, the term "cholesterol lowering" is actually a medical claim, and until recently the FDA had only limited jurisdiction over such labeling. As a result, in the previous few years, 40 percent of new food products introduced to the marketplace made favorable health statements of one sort or another. Fortunately, new food labeling laws forbid unverified medical claims.

Insoluble fiber is found in bran, vegetables, and fruits. Many fruits, vegetables, legumes, and cereal products also contain *soluble* fiber. Among these are oat bran, rice bran, and corn bran. Bran products, eaten in hopes of lowering cholesterol, can be tricky however. Beware of cereals processed with considerable amouns of fat, some of it saturated and likely to *raise* blood cholesterol. For example, Kellogg's Cracklin' Oat Bran gets 30 percent of its calories from fat, more than a third of it saturated.*

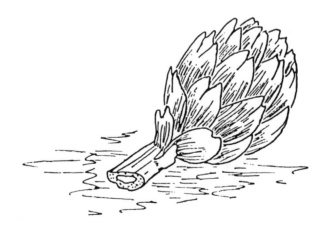

---

*Each 110 calorie serving contains 4g of fat; at 9 calories per gram this translates to 36 calories of fat, which represents 33% of total calories.

	Low Fiber	Medium Fiber	High Fiber
CEREALS	Cream of rice Cream of wheat Farina Puffed rice White rice	Oatmeal Shredded wheat Cornflakes Granola Brown rice Barley	Bran (all kinds) Bran flakes
BREAD	White Italian French Rye	Whole wheat Pumpernickel (made of whole grain flour)	
VEGETABLES	Strained juice	Lettuce Onions Snap beans Carrots Tomatoes Peppers Spinach	Artichokes Most beans Lentils Peas Chickpeas Broccoli Corn
FRUITS	Strained juice	Bananas Melons Applesauce Plums Peaches Grapes Citrus fruit Cherries	Berries Whole apples Whole pears Figs Dates Prunes
NUTS		Peanuts Almonds Walnuts	Brazil nuts Coconuts

Representative items in several food groups are listed above according to relative fiber content.

Current guidelines recommend 25 gm of fiber daily; that is slightly less than an ounce. A typical western diet contains about ½ ounce, half of it from legumes and vegetables, the other half from cereals and fruits. In less industrialized regions, where foods are not highly processed, adults may consume 4 ounces a day or more.

An inadequate intake of fiber in western countries is blamed for various "diseases of civilization," chiefly affecting the bowel. This suspicion is not new. The Greek physician Hippocrates advised that the bran be left in meal (flour) to help bowel function.

An excessive amount of fiber, however, can cause rumbling, bloating, and diarrhea and it may also interfere with the absorption of vitamins and some important minerals. The wisest course is to eat a balanced diet that includes, among other things, fresh fruits, vegetables, and whole-grain cereal products.

LOW-RESIDUE AND BLAND DIETS

A low-residue diet eliminates foods high in fiber. A bland diet is similar to a low-residue diet, but it is also restricted with regard to spices. These diets are designed to soothe the intestinal tract and to lighten the digestive workload. Transit through the bowel is slowed; stools are small and infrequent.

Shown below are lists of foods appropriate and inappropriate for such diets.

Foods Permitted in Low-Residue and Bland Diets
Precooked or cooked fine cereals
Noodles and pasta
White bread
Cream soups
Milk, cream, butter, cottage and cream cheese, yogurt
Margarine, oil
Eggs (not fried)
Potatoes (skinned and not fried)
Strained or chopped sweet potatoes, squash, carrots
Bananas, cooked fruit without skins
Strained fruit juices
Ground meat, cooked, not fried
Ice cream, fruit gelatin, custard, pudding

Foods Not Allowed
Whole grain breads and cereals
Meat extract or stock
Processed meats and cheeses
Raw vegetables
Cooked cabbage, corn, and legumes

Raw fruit, except bananas
Strong spices and flavorings
Nuts
Tea, coffee, and carbonated drinks
Any form of alcohol

CEREAL GRAINS

This is a loosely defined group of a number of very important food plants. Technically, most of these crops are actually the seeds of grasses, but one, buckwheat, is a fruit. All are high in carbohydrates. Protein and fat contents vary, and so does the amount of bran. *Bran* is the seed covering of cereal plants. It is largely indigestible, but serves as a source of fiber and some B vitamins.

Brief descriptions of various plants are given below in alphabetical order. If importance were used as the ranking criterion, corn, wheat, and rice would head the list.

Amaranth: a high-protein designer grain, first cultivated by the Aztecs.

Barley: probably the most ancient cultivated cereal grain, with evidence of prehistoric use in China and Egypt. Since Greek and Roman times it has been grown exten- 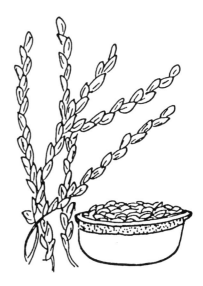 sively as a source of food and animal feed, and for the production of liquor. *Barley corn* is a grain of barley. *Pearl barley* has had all outer layers removed from the grain.

Barley and some other grains can be subjected to a special process that produces malt. Malt is used in beer-making and also in some foods and drugs.

Buckwheat: a plant that produces kernels known as *groats*. Compared to other crops, groats are rich in amino acids. Roasted groats are sold as *kasha.* Buckwheat is especially important in poor farming areas, because it is very hardy and can be grown in poor soil.

Corn: "the American grain," *maize,* introduced to Europe by Spaniards returning from New World conquests; it is now an invaluable crop worldwide for food, animal fodder, and for the manufacture of corn oil, corn syrup (a major commercial sweetener), cornstarch, dextrose, and many other food and nonfood products. (The Americas also gave the world potatoes, tomatoes, peppers, and cocoa.)

Cornmeal (polenta) consists of ground whole kernels of corn. *Hominy* is made of hulled kernels. (Native Americans did the hulling by soaking corn in a weak lye solution.) Hominy can then be ground to produce *grits.*

Bourbon is distilled from a mash that is at least 50 percent corn; corn whiskey contains at least 80 percent corn mash.

Emmer: a hardy European grain closely related to wheat.

Millet: one of the oldest of grains, cultivated for over 4,000 years. A tall grass, carrying small seeds, millet grows fast and resists drought. It is still the food staple of India, and is common in underdeveloped areas of Asia and Africa. The protein content of millet is lower than that of wheat.

Oats: a grain grown in temperate and cool climates all over the world. It is used for dry and cooked cereals, and provides important animal fodder that is relatively high in protein, minerals, and vitamins. Oat bran supplies water soluble fiber, as opposed to unprocessed wheat bran, which is insoluble.

Quinoa: the sacred mother grain of the Incas, still used widely in the Andes. It is high in protein. Quinoa is now increasingly cultivated in the United States, where a similar plant, known as lamb's quarters, has long grown wild.

Rice: known for 9,000 years, and cultivated for almost that long. Rice is the main dietary staple of more people than any other food. Protein content is relatively low.

More than 7,000 varieties have been developed. Western countries prefer *long grain* rice. *Short grain,* used in Far Eastern countries, is more glutinous or sticky. (Glutinous does not mean that it contains gluten.) Sticky rice is the main component of sushi. *Brown* or *unpolished* rice has more vitamins and fiber than polished rice, because the bran remains (after the husk has been removed). *Converted rice* is processed to retain much of the fiber and nutrients. *Instant rice* is pre-cooked, and is the least nutritious. Several foreign grown varieties of rice are now available in the United States in addition to Far Eastern types, among them *Arborio,* a short-grain creamy rice from Italy, and *Basmati,* an aromatic white or brown long-grain variety from India.

Sake and other alcoholic beverages are made from rice.

Rye: a grain closely related to wheat, most commonly grown in northern Europe and other cool climates. Because rye does not contain much gluten, it produces a heavy, dense bread. In the United States wheat flour is usually mixed with it to produce a lighter color and tex-ture.

Rye can be fermented to make whiskey.

Sorghum: a plant that resembles corn in appearance. It is used as a forage plant and also for food in the United States, India, China, and Africa. Some varieties yield a syrup.

Triticale: a hybrid between wheat and rye that has a high protein con-tent.

Wheat: among the world's largest food crops, used primarily for making flour. Wheat was first grown in the Nile valley at least 7,000 years ago. About a dozen species and literally thousands of varieties are cultivated, depending on climate, soil, intended use, pest resistance, lo-cal disease, and regional prefer-ence.

Common wheat, a species that includes numerous varieties, is the favorite grain for bread-making, because it contains in its kernel a large quantity of gluten, which helps to make dough rise and gives bread its characteristic texture. Va-rieties of the *durum* species are used in pasta-making, because they allow macaroni products to hold up with cooking. *Semolina* is a purified component of durum. *Graham* flour is whole wheat flour. *Cracked wheat* is wheat that has been dried, and then cracked and ground. *Bulgur wheat* is first cooked, then dried and ground. *Wheat berries* are unprocessed wheat kernels. *Wheat germ,* a part of each wheat kernel, is a substance rich in vitamin E and manganese.

Wheat is used to make beer and whiskey.

Wild rice: the seeds of a water grass first harvested by Native Americans, now grown commercially.

GLUTEN

Gluten is an insoluble *protein* ingredient of most grains, including wheat, rye, oats, barley, and buckwheat. It is the material that gives elasticity to dough. In certain disorders of intestinal absorption, gluten must be restricted.

Foods to be avoided in a gluten-restricted diet
Noodles and pasta
Most commercial baked goods
Wheat, rye, oat, barley, and buckwheat cereals
Processed meats and cheeses
Gravies, sauces, and soups made with flour
Breadings and stuffings
Most ice creams
Cocoa mix, malted milk, most syrups
Beer, ale, whiskey

Foods that are permitted
Plain vegetables, fruits, and fruit juices
Potatoes and rice
Rice and corn cereals
Baked goods made with potato, rice, corn, or soy flour
Milk, natural cheese, eggs, butter
Oil, margarine
Meat, fowl, fish, shellfish
Gelatin, sherbet
Honey, jam, jelly, sugar
Coffee, tea, carbonated drinks

Several companies make gluten-free food products, and these are labeled as such.

OXALIC ACID (OXALATE)

Oxalic acid is a component of many plants. The following food items contain considerable quantities of oxalate.

VEGETABLES AND HERBS	Purslane, pokeweed, sorrel, rhubarb, beets, spinach, peppers, parsley, scallions, celery, carrots, artichoke, yams, okra, rhubarb
FRUITS	Plums, red grapes, berries, figs, oranges
MISCELLANEOUS	Instant coffee, cocoa, cola drinks, beer, pecans, peanuts, peanut butter

Even though it is a naturally occurring substance, oxalic acid is potentially harmful. It is present at such low concentrations, however, that it presents no risk of toxicity to healthy individuals when eaten in conventional food portions. When taken in very large quantities, or in certain medical conditions, it can hamper the absorption of important minerals, particularly calcium and magnesium, by combining with them and tying them into unusable oxalate salts.

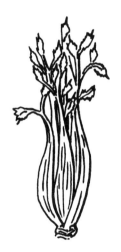

Rare cases of itching and burning have been attributed to an oxalate intolerance.

FASCINATING FACTS ABOUT CARBOHYDRATES

- Sugar is no more likely to cause tooth decay than other carbohydrates. What matters is how much sticks to the teeth over a period of time.
- "Complex carbohydrates" are foods whose chief component is a form of starch. This includes cereals, breads, pasta, rice, and potatoes. Fruits and vegetables are primarily complex carbohydrates

too, but they usually also contain a significant amount of fiber and water. Complex carbohydrates are much in fashion now, just as high-protein foods were in previous decades.

- "Wheat flour" on a label does not mean whole wheat flour. Bread marked "100 percent whole wheat" is made of whole wheat flour, but the term "whole wheat bread" means very little, unless whole wheat flour is the first listed ingredient. If whole wheat flour is not the main flour used, the dark color of wheat bread usually comes from caramel or molasses, and the bread is not nutritionally superior to white bread.
- Ounce for ounce, prunes have two-thirds the calories of cornflakes and four-and-a-half times as much fiber.
- Potatoes often have fewer calories than their various embellishments. A medium baked potato, for instance, provides 95 calories, while that tablespoon of butter provides 108.
- Bran muffins get about 40 percent of their calories from fat.

CHAPTER 3

The Many Faces of Fat

Fats are a major concern today to consumers, nutritionists, basic scientists, and food providers. This chapter is slightly technical in part, for those who want to understand the terms a little more fully.

Fat is the most concentrated source of calories, furnishing more than twice as much energy per unit weight as protein or carbohydrate. Foods with a fat content of 20 to 30 percent, such as certain meats, cold cuts, and cheeses, actually derive more than half their calories from fat. For example, American cheese contains 30 percent fat by weight, but fat provides 73 percent of the calories.

The average American gets between 35 and 40 percent of his calories from fat. Current thinking holds that it should be no more than 30 percent. A 1,700 calorie diet, for example, should contain no more than two ounces of fat; this includes the fat within the food product, fat used in cooking, and fat added to food, such as salad oil. An ounce of pure fat provides 255 calories, so that two ounces would supply 510 calories or 30 percent of the daily caloric intake.

HIGH-FAT FOODS

Listed below are a few selected foods that derive a large part of their calories from fat.

	Approximate Percentage of Calories from Fat
Butter	100
Margarine	100
Oil	100
Vegetable shortening	100
Mayonnaise	99
Heavy cream	97
Macadamia nuts	94
Cream cheese	90
Light cream	90
Salad dressing (avg.)	90
Greek olives	89
Sour cream	86
Beef frankfurter	82
Baking chocolate	77
Half & half	77
Peanuts and peanut butter	76
Sunflower seeds	76
American cheese	76
Cheddar cheese	74
Avocado	72
Chicken frankfurter	68
Liquid non dairy creamer	68
T-bone steak, trimmed	65
Egg	64
Pork loin	64
Vanilla ice cream (16% fat)	61
Partially defatted peanuts	60
Cream of mushroom soup (with milk)	60
Raised doughnut	58
Pie crust	57
Potato chips	57
Croissant	55
Milk chocolate	54
Tofu (soybean curd)	53
Ritz cracker	50
Granola	50

FAST FOODS AND SNACK FOODS

The following list gives the approximate caloric value and the number of calories provided by fat in some common fast foods and snack foods.

	Total Calories	Calories from Fat	Percent Calories from Fat
HAMBURGERS			
Burger King	260	90	35
Burger King Whopper	630	351	56
McDonald's	255	81	32
McDonald's Big Mac	500	234	47
Wendy's	350	135	39
Wendy's double cheeseburger	800	432	54
FISH SANDWICHES			
Burger King BK Big Fish	720	387	54
McDonald's Filet-O-Fish	370	162	44
CHICKEN SANDWICHES			
Burger King Chicken	700	387	55
KFC Colonel's Chicken	482	243	50
McDonald's McChicken	470	225	48
Wendy's Breaded Chicken	450	180	40
CHICKEN NUGGETS—6 pieces			
Burger King Chicken Tenders	250	108	43
KFC Kentucky Nuggets	284	162	57
McDonald's Chicken McNuggets	270	135	50
ROAST BEEF SANDWICHES			
Arby's	383	162	42
Hardee's	280	99	35
FRENCH FRIES medium			
Burger King	400	180	45
McDonald's	320	153	48
Wendy's	340	153	45
MEXICAN FOOD			
Taco Bell Beef Burrito	466	189	41
Taco Bell Salad with Shell	905	560	62
Wendy's Chili	230	72	31
PIZZA			
Celeste ¼ frozen deluxe	365	168	46
Domino's two slices, deep dish	560	216	39
Pizza Hut, two slices, thin	506	162	32
CHIPS AND LOW FAT CHIPS, 1 oz			
Fritos corn chips	155	87	56
Lay's potato chips	149	86	57
Wise tortilla chips	150	70	47
Guiltless Gourmet nachos	110	9	8
Snack Appeal crisps	110	14	12

	Total Calories	Calories from Fat	Percent Calories from Fat
FROZEN DESSERT			
Haagen-Dazs ice cream, 4 oz	270	153	57
Haagen-Dazs frozen yogurt 4 oz	220	81	37
Toffuti, 4 oz	230	126	55
Elan frozen yogurt, 4 oz	125	27	22
Tuscan yogurt pop	130	63	48
Tofulite chocolate bar	240	135	56
JELL-O vanilla pudding pop	70	18	26
Weight Watchers sandwich bar	150	27	18
Vitari frozen dessert	80	0	0
Dairy Queen banana split	540	35	25
Dairy Queen large cone	390	90	26
COOKIES — 1 piece			
Keebler Chips Ahoy	80	45	56
Nabisco Fig Newton	60	9	15
Nabisco fat free Fig Newton	70	0	0
Pepperidge Farm granola cookie	159	69	41
SWEETS and NUTS, 1 oz			
Hershey milk chocolate	157	83	53
Oh Henry!	139	64	46
Carob bar	140	68	49
Roasted peanuts	170	126	74
Roasted peanuts, defatted	154	90	58

FATS AND FATTY ACIDS

Total fat is not the only factor. Fats differ in their health effects. It is recommended that the total fat allowance be divided equally among saturated, monounsaturated, and polyunsaturated fatty acids, with each of the three supplying about 10 percent of total calories.

Saturated fatty acids provide the fats in the diet that have been linked to elevated blood cholesterol and to damaging effects on blood vessels, including those that supply the heart and brain. "Saturated" means that the fatty acid molecule holds all the hydrogen it can.

"Hydrogenation" (often seen on a label) is a process that creates a type of fat not found in nature. The process is used to make an oil solid

at room temperature, such as margarine and vegetable shortening, and also to make products more stable (to increase their "shelf life"). When vegetable oils are hydrogenated, they form *trans fatty acids*. These trans fats behave like saturated fats in their effect on the lipid profile.

Fats are usually mixtures of several different fatty acids and fatty acid *types*. As a general rule, the more saturated a fat product is, the more likely it will be solid at room temperature, and also the more stable on heating and prolonged storage. Some fats, such as soybean oil, undergo a degree of hydrogenation during heating. For this reason soybean oil is often sold mixed with corn oil, or it is deliberately partly hydrogenated and then purified; this makes it more suitable for cooking and also retards rancidity.

Saturated fatty acids themselves appear to differ in their effect on blood cholesterol levels. Myristic acid, particularly prominent in butter fat and tropical oils, raises cholesterol more than other acids.

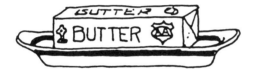

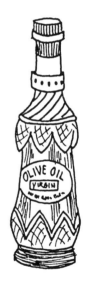

Stearic acid, found especially in beef and chocolate, may by itself actually lower cholesterol, but unfortunately is present in these foods along with less favorable saturated fatty acids.

Monounsaturated fatty acids have one double bond capable of absorbing an additional hydrogen atom. These fatty acids tend to produce a more favorable blood cholesterol profile, namely a lower cholesterol and a higher HDL/LDL ratio.* Population studies also suggest that monounsaturates help with control of blood sugar in diabetics.

Polyunsaturated fatty acids have two or more double bonds that provide available sites for additional atoms. They too play a role in lowering cholesterol and blood sugar. Some of them, moreover, are essen-

---

*These terms are defined in the Lipoprotein section

tial for adequate nutrition; the human body cannot produce them, and they must be included in the diet. (Fats are found in so many varieties of foods, however, including many fruits and vegetables, that this rarely presents a problem.)

Their good reputation notwithstanding, polyunsaturated fatty acids are not necessarily the unqualified best choice of fat. Monounsaturated fatty acids invite fewer free radicals* upon heating than do the polyunsaturated fatty acids, and this is in their favor. Monounsaturated oils, such as olive oil, may turn out to be the best choice for cooking, but the jury is still out.

Shown below, in simplified diagram form, are prototypes of fatty acid "chains." Actually, the chains can be much longer. Marine polyunsaturates have more than 18 carbon atoms; 25 to 30 percent of the chains have as many as 20 or 22 carbons, and as many as 6 double bonds, indicating a high degree of unsaturation. Mammalian and most vegetable fats have fewer long chains and fewer double bonds, and the double bonds occur at different sites.

Saturated fatty acids have no double carbon-carbon bonds; that is, the carbon atoms (C) are connected to each other with single bonds (-).

$$\text{---}\overset{\overset{\text{H}}{|}}{\underset{\underset{\text{H}}{|}}{\text{C}}}\text{-}\overset{\overset{\text{H}}{|}}{\underset{\underset{\text{H}}{|}}{\text{C}}}\text{-}\overset{\overset{\text{H}}{|}}{\underset{\underset{\text{H}}{|}}{\text{C}}}\text{-}\overset{\overset{\text{H}}{|}}{\underset{\underset{\text{H}}{|}}{\text{C}}}\text{-}\text{---}$$

Monounsaturated fatty acids have one double bond (=) where hydrogen atoms (H) could otherwise be attached.

$$\text{---}\overset{\overset{\text{H}}{|}}{\underset{\underset{\text{H}}{|}}{\text{C}}}\text{-}\overset{\overset{\text{H}}{|}}{\underset{\underset{\text{H}}{|}}{\text{C}}}\text{-}\overset{\overset{\text{H}}{|}}{\text{C}}\text{=}\overset{\overset{\text{H}}{|}}{\text{C}}\text{-}\overset{\overset{\text{H}}{|}}{\underset{\underset{\text{H}}{|}}{\text{C}}}\text{-}\overset{\overset{\text{H}}{|}}{\underset{\underset{\text{H}}{|}}{\text{C}}}\text{-}\text{---}$$

Polyunsaturated fatty acids have two or more double bonds.

$$\text{---}\overset{\overset{\text{H}}{|}}{\underset{\underset{\text{H}}{|}}{\text{C}}}\text{-}\overset{\overset{\text{H}}{|}}{\text{C}}\text{=}\overset{\overset{\text{H}}{|}}{\text{C}}\text{-}\overset{\overset{\text{H}}{|}}{\underset{\underset{\text{H}}{|}}{\text{C}}}\text{-}\overset{\overset{\text{H}}{|}}{\text{C}}\text{=}\overset{\overset{\text{H}}{|}}{\text{C}}\text{-}\overset{\overset{\text{H}}{|}}{\underset{\underset{\text{H}}{|}}{\text{C}}}\text{-}\text{---}$$

For those interested in technical details: Fatty acids can also be described with monograms which indicate the length of the carbon chain, the number of double bonds, and the location of the first of these double bonds from the end of the chain. For example, C18:2n-6 means an 18-carbon chain with 2 double bonds, the first of them at the 6th carbon (the n-6 or omega-6 position). Fish oils are n-3 or omega-3 fatty acids.

---

*See Free Radicals and Antioxidants

CHOLESTEROL AND SATURATED FAT

Cholesterol is not a fatty acid, and it cannot be said to provide calories. It is a waxy substance that is a component of all animal tissue (except egg white), and all meat and dairy products. In our bodies it plays a vital role with regard to cell structure and stability. It is also a necessary building block for a number of hormones.

Ordinarily about a third of the body's cholesterol comes from food, the rest is made by our own cells, chiefly in the liver. After infancy no cholesterol needs to be included in the diet because the body produces all it needs.

We read and hear a great deal about cholesterol because studies have shown that there is an association between high levels of cholesterol *in the blood* and the probability of a heart attack and other medical problems. It is important, however, not to confuse cholesterol in the blood with the cholesterol that we eat. This is a very important point!

Cholesterol in food does have an impact on blood cholesterol, but it is only one of many factors, and not the most significant one. Saturated fats are more damaging. It is also true that cholesterol-rich foods are often high in saturated fat as well.

Current thinking holds that we should limit our cholesterol intake to about 300 mg a day; and, as stated, earlier, no more than 10 percent of our calories should come from saturated fatty acids. Eating saturated fats is more apt to raise the blood cholesterol than will eating cholesterol itself. (A definition of saturated fat is found in the section on fats and fatty acids.)

Unlike cholesterol, saturated fats may be of animal or vegetable origin; cholesterol is found *only* in animal products.

There is great variation in the saturated fat content of meat, depending on the amount of visible fat and the marbling of the meat. (The choicest, most tender cuts often contain the most marbling, and therefore the most fat.)

Cholesterol is *invisible* and is found even in lean muscle tissue. That pertains not only to meat and poultry, but also to fish and shellfish. The nutritionally important differences between beef and veal, or between meat, poultry, and seafood, lie chiefly in their saturated fat content, rather than in the amount of cholesterol they contain.

Saturated Fat and Cholesterol Content in Comparable Portions of Meat, Poultry and Seafood

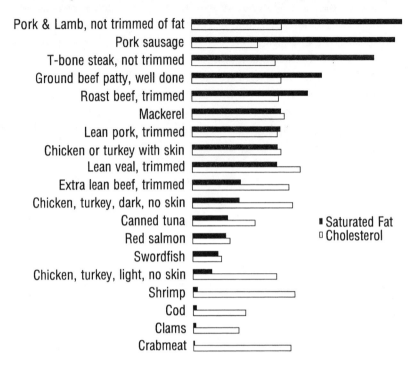

It is hard to say what a "normal" cholesterol is. For one thing we must not confuse "normal" with "average," because the average in western society is now considered too high; and for another, what is usually measured is "total" cholesterol, which is not necessarily the most significant assessment. (This is discussed further under "Lipoproteins.") Broadly speaking, and without regard to age or sex or ever-changing opinions and guidelines, it is best to aim for a total blood cholesterol below 200 mg percent.

Listed below are average portions of some common food items, their caloric value (Cal), the number of calories provided by *saturated* fat (Sat Fat Cal), and the cholesterol content (Chol). All values are approximate. No allowances are made for fat that is added in cooking or serving.

To reiterate current guidelines: limiting saturated fat intake is more meaningful than limiting cholesterol. Saturated fat calories should not exceed one tenth of total calories, and therefore should range from 100 to 300 calories daily, depending on one's total caloric requirement. One ounce of any kind of fat supplies about 250 calories.

	Cal	Sat Fat Cal	Chol (mg)
MEAT: 3.5 oz (100 gms) cooked weight			
Beef, extra lean, trimmed of fat	190	25	90
Ground beef patty	280	65	90
Roast beef, trimmed of visible fat	242	58	87
T-bone steak, "choice," not trimmed	330	92	84
Beef liver	161	17	420
Veal rump roast, lean only	156	42	118
Veal blade (breast), not trimmed	250	90	90
Lamb leg roast, lean only	191	27	99
Lamb rib chop meat, not trimmed	344	120	90
Pork tenderloin, lean only	166	15	80
Pork loin, lean only	240	45	89
Pork loin chop meat, not trimmed	390	103	90
Ham, cured, boneless	215	32	92
Pork sausage	389	100	68
Chicken or turkey, light, no skin	170	10	84
Chicken or turkey, dark, no skin	194	24	95
Chicken or turkey with skin (avg)	244	42	90
Chicken liver	205	16	550
Brains	100	19	1,960
PROCESSED MEAT: 2 oz (58 gms)			
Bologna (2 or 3 slices)	178	60	32
Boiled ham, very lean, 2 slices	78	10	26
Turkey bologna	140	26	57
Turkey ham	73	9	34
Liverwurst	190	55	88
Salami, dry hard (5 or 6 slices)	244	63	48
Frankfurter, beef and/or pork	185	56	29
Frankfurter, chicken or turkey	140	29	55
FISH AND SHELLFISH, 3.5 oz (100 gms)			
Caviar	260	90	300
Clams	120	2	47
Cod	105	2	55

	Cal	Sat Fat Cal	Chol (mg)
Crabmeat	102	2	100
Haddock	80	2	60
Halibut	100	4	50
Lobster	92	1	85
Mackerel	198	45	93
Oysters	66	0	50
Salmon	185	30	36
Shrimp	49	1	112
Swordfish	155	13	30
Tuna, canned in oil	198	18	65

DAIRY PRODUCTS, EGGS AND SUBSTITUTES

	Cal	Sat Fat Cal	Chol (mg)
Whole milk, 3½% butterfat, 8 oz.	150	46	33
Skim milk, 8 oz	86	3	5
Heavy cream, 1 oz	100	60	40
Evaporated milk, 1 oz	42	13	10
Non-dairy creamer, soybean oil, 1 oz	40	5	0
Non-dairy creamer, tropical oil, 1 oz	40	25	0
Butter, 1 tbs	108	68	32
Margarine, corn oil stick, 1 tbs	108	22	0
Country Crock, 1 tbs	60	14	0
Ice cream, 16% fat, ½ cup	175	66	44
Ice cream, 10% fat, ½ cup	135	40	30
Yogurt, whole milk, 8 oz	148	43	29
Yogurt, low fat, 8 oz	130	21	14
Cottage cheese, ½ cup	117	29	24
Cottage cheese, 1% butterfat, ½ cup	82	6	12
Cream cheese, cheddar, blue, 2 oz	230	109	62
Cream cheese, whipped, light	140	72	40
American, Swiss, Parmesan, 2 oz	180	72	50
American non-fat (Kraft Free)	90	0	10
Eggs, 2 large	158	31	426
Eggbeaters, equivalent of 2 eggs	50	0	0
Tofutti Egg Watchers, 2 eggs	100	5	0
Scramblers, equivalent of 2 eggs	120	18	0
Egg yolks, 2 large	125	31	426
Egg whites, 2 large	33	0	0

FATS, OILS, DRESSINGS and SPREADS, 1 tbs

	Cal	Sat Fat Cal	Chol (mg)
Lard	116	45	15
Beef tallow	116	58	14
Cod-liver oil	120	10	81
Coconut oil	120	106	0

	Cal	Sat Fat Cal	Chol (mg)
Other oils—(see Different Oils . . .)	120		
Vegetable shortening	106	29	0
Non-stick spray (1½ seconds)	8	2	0
Oil/vinegar dressing	70	9	0
Hollandaise and similar sauces	45	24	12
Gravy, canned	12	2	1
Mayonnaise	100	18	5
Peanut butter	94	14	0
Jam or jelly	55	0	0

VEGETABLES, FRUITS and NUTS

Vegetable products do not contain cholesterol. Most fruits and vegetables are also *fat* free; some that are *not* are listed below.

Avocado, ½ large	230	32	0
Banana, medium	105	2	0
Chickpeas, 4 oz, canned	205	4	0
Coconut meat, 1 oz	102	78	0
Olives, 2 oz (10–12 large)	110	9	0
Peanuts, 1 oz	170	28	0
Pumpkin seeds, 1 oz	157	21	0
Tofu, 4 oz	85	7	0
Wheat germ, 1 oz	108	5	0

BAKED GOODS, CEREALS, PASTA and SWEETS

Baked goods vary widely, depending on inclusion of eggs and milk, as well as type and quantity of fat. Estimates are given.

Bagel	200	3	0
Bread, white or whole wheat, 1 slice	70	3	1
Biscuit, 1 oz, from mix	93	5	2
Biscuit, 1 oz, lard or solid shortening	103	6	15
Corn muffin	145	14	23
Croissant, large	235	32	13
English muffin	140	3	0
Hamburger or hot dog bun	115	5	1
Popover	112	15	71
Ritz crackers, 5 pieces	90	12	3
Saltines, 5 pieces	65	4	0
Corn flakes, 1 cup (0.8 oz)	94	0	0
Granola, 1 cup	505	52	0
Oatmeal, ¾ cup (1 oz dry)	108	3	0
Spaghetti, cooked, 1 cup	190	2	0
Egg noodles, cooked, 1 cup	160	6	50
Angel food cake, slice	125	0	0

	Cal	Sat Fat Cal	Chol (mg)
Chocolate chip cookie	46	12	9
Chocolate cake with icing, 3 oz	310	65	36
Doughnut, plain	210	24	20
Fruit cake	167	22	27
Lemon meringue pie, ⅙ of 9″ pie	355	39	143
Sponge cake, 3 oz	235	14	201
Milk chocolate, 1 oz	142	54	6

THE DIFFERENT OILS AND FATS

The table below shows the fatty acid content of the various familiar fats and oils and indicates which ones contain cholesterol.

	SFA	MONO	PUFA	
	(as percent of total fat)			
OILS				
Canola oil	6	62	32	Lowest in SFA
Coconut oil	84	11	1	Highest in SFA
Cod-liver oil	8	49	37	X
Corn oil	13	25	62	
Cottonseed oil	27	19	54	
Olive oil	13	76	9	Highest in MONO
Palm kernel oil	79	16	2	
Palm oil	48	40	9	Very High in SFA
Peanut oil	17	50	32	SFA
Safflower oil	10	14	75	
Sesame oil	14	42	43	
Soybean oil	16	23	61	Highest in PUFA
Sunflower oil	12	19	68	
Walnut oil	9	18	73	
Wheat germ oil	29	18	53	
FATS				
Beef fat	50	46	4	X
Butter	60	36	4	X
Chicken fat	30	49	21	X
Lard (pork fat)	39	50	11	X
Margarine (average)	19	53	27	
Vegetable shortening	29	44	27	

(**SFA** saturated fatty acids; **MONO** monounsaturated fatty acids; **PUFA** polyunsaturated fatty acids; **X** contains cholesterol

Which one of the oils is recommended most highly? Canola oil (made from rapeseed) is healthy, but imparts an unpleasant taste when used for frying. Olive oil is tried and true, versatile, comes in different grades and varieties, but is more expensive. Peanut oil is excellent for frying, but, when used in salads, gives them its own distinct flavor. Sunflower oil, safflower oil (made from a thistle plant) and corn oil are good all-round selections, though not outstanding in any category. Cottonseed oil is more saturated than others, but excellent for frying, and inexpensive. The final selection rests with the consumer.

LIPOPROTEINS

Since fats will not dissolve in blood, which is a watery substance, they must be transported through the bloodstream wrapped in other compounds. These compounds are the lipoproteins, complex combinations of proteins and fats. Among them are the high density lipoproteins (HDL), low density lipoproteins (LDL), and very low density lipoproteins (VLDL). (The term density, as in high or low density, is related to the laboratory method used in lipoprotein testing.) In accordance with their different structures, lipoproteins carry different proportions of cholesterol and triglycerides, and they have different functions. Triglycerides are carried mainly by VLDL and comprise the greatest part of that molecule. About two-thirds of all cholesterol is transported by LDL.

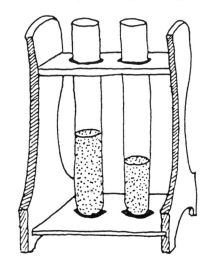

Stated in simplified terms, LDL and VLDL are bad because they encourage deposition of fatty material in the walls of blood vessels and therefore contribute to the risk of heart disease and stroke. HDL is good because it removes cholesterol from tissues, mostly to be disposed of by the liver. Unfortunately HDLs do not occur as such in foods; they must be manufactured by the body, rather than eaten. (This is equally true of the other lipoprotein fractions.) Exercise, female hormones, and moderate alcohol consumption all contribute to raising HDL.

Lipoprotein testing has assumed an important role in recent years. Many physicians and scientists now think that, for the purpose of assessing cardiovascular risk, measuring total cholesterol (TC) is not nearly as revealing as measuring lipoprotein fractions. A low or normal TC composed mainly of LDL-cholesterol may be more ominous than a TC that is slightly elevated but has a high HDL-cholesterol portion. In rural societies of South America and the Far East, where fat consumption is low, there is not much cardiovascular disease, even though average HDLs are low. But in industrialized countries it appears that the ratios as well as the absolute numbers are significant in risk assessment. Of all the tests related to cholesterol, the TC/HDL ratio may be the best marker in risk assessment.

Desirable values are different for men and women and for different ages. Nevertheless, the values shown below may be useful, if they are taken as approximations rather than firm guidelines. They apply to adults only.

Lab Test	Desirable Value
TC	less than 200 mg %*
LDL	less than 100 mg %
HDL	more than 45 mg %
TC/HDL	less than 4.5 mg %
Triglycerides	less than 160 mg %

TRIGLYCERIDES

Triglycerides are fatty substances normally present in the blood. They are carried as part of the lipoprotein molecule, chiefly on VLDL (see Lipoproteins). There is uncertainty about the significance of slightly elevated triglycerides; it may or may not represent a risk factor for heart disease in otherwise healthy people. Very high triglycerides indicate an inborn abnormality, or they reflect an underlying illness. In

---

*A mg % is a thousandth of a percent of a blood sample or one part in a hundred thousand

any event, marked elevation does indeed pose a threat, and medical intervention is advisable.

Best values are below 160 mg percent with blood drawn in the fasting state.

FISH AND FISH OIL

Although the Inuit (Eskimos) eat a diet high in animal fat and cholesterol and low in vegetables and vegetable fats, they have a lower rate of heart disease than other North Americans whose average diet consists of less fat and more carbohydrates. Current thinking attributes this to the *type* of fat found in fish, seal, and whale meat. Even though this flesh is of animal origin, and therefore contains cholesterol, it is indirectly derived from cold-water plants and remains liquid at very low temperatures. Not surprisingly, it is the fish from the coldest waters (particularly the North Atlantic) that is richest in these fats.

The substances most specifically involved are two polyunsaturated so-called omega-3 fatty acids, EPA and DHA (full names: eicosopentaenoic acid and docosahexaenoic acid). The best source of omega-3 fatty acids are the oilier fish such as mackerel, herring, sardines, salmon, sturgeon, and carp.

The benefits of omega-3 fatty acids appear to be related to several effects: they reduce the stickiness of blood (by changing blood platelet activity in various ways), they lower cholesterol and triglycerides in the blood, and they improve the ratio between "good" cholesterol (HDL) and "bad" cholesterol (LDL). The first of these effects is probably the most important; however, it is also the one that should mitigate against excessive intake of these fatty acids, since adequate platelet activity is required to prevent abnormal bleeding.

Omega-3 fatty acids are also reported to protect cigarette smokers against serious chronic lung disease, and to reduce high blood pressure, but this needs to be substantiated.

It must be remembered that, like other animal products, seafood contains cholesterol. This is true also of fish oils; a tablespoon of cod liver oil contains more than twice as much cholesterol as a tablespoon of butter. Fish oil supplements have not been fully validated as good substitutes for real fish. They should be used only under medical supervision.

Incidentally, some vegetables also contain omega-3 fatty acids, but these differ from marine fatty acids in molecule size. Their value in the diet has not been determined. The richest plant source is purslane, a vegetable most commonly used in the eastern Mediterranean. Vegetable oils are primarily omega-6 fatty acids, but recent work suggests that some of them, especially soybean oil, can be partly converted by the body to the omega-3 variety.

$$H-\underset{\underset{H}{|}}{\overset{\overset{H}{|}}{C}}-\underset{\underset{H}{|}}{\overset{\overset{H}{|}}{C}}-\overset{\overset{H}{|}}{C}=\overset{\overset{H}{|}}{C}-\underset{\underset{H}{|}}{\overset{\overset{H}{|}}{C}}-\cdots$$

omega-3 position

$$H-\underset{\underset{H}{|}}{\overset{\overset{H}{|}}{C}}-\underset{\underset{H}{|}}{\overset{\overset{H}{|}}{C}}-\underset{\underset{H}{|}}{\overset{\overset{H}{|}}{C}}-\underset{\underset{H}{|}}{\overset{\overset{H}{|}}{C}}-\underset{\underset{H}{|}}{\overset{\overset{H}{|}}{C}}-\overset{\overset{H}{|}}{C}=\overset{\overset{H}{|}}{C}-\underset{\underset{H}{|}}{\overset{\overset{H}{|}}{C}}-\cdots$$

omega-6 position

At present the average American outside Alaska consumes at least ten times as much meat as fish.

LECITHIN

Lecithins are sticky waxy substances found in cells throughout the body. Lecithin is particularly important in the structure of nerve tissue and its coverings.

Lecithins mix readily with water and can change the physical texture of fat by homogenizing it into a more liquid state. This property is utilized not only in the body, but also commercially in the manufacture of ice cream, chocolate, baked goods, and many other foods.

When produced as a health food supplement, lecithin is usually an extract of soybeans. It may also be derived from other fat sources such as egg yolks and milk. As a nutritional supplement, lecithin has been advocated in the treatment of memory loss, as well as for several specific neurologic and psychiatric illnesses. It has also been recommended for the prevention of hardening of the arteries and high blood pressure, and particularly for lowering blood cholesterol. None of these claims has ever been substantiated in controlled studies. The one thing lecithin supplements actually do is add calories to the diet.

Estimated daily requirement: not known
Estimated average daily intake: 10 gm
Richest sources: Soybeans
Legumes
Egg yolks
Brains

There are no known lecithin-deficiency symptoms in humans.
Toxic effects of lecithin have not been proved, but there have been reports of depression, headaches, gastrointestinal symptoms, and rash when lecithin supplements exceeded 30 grams daily.

CHOLINE

Choline is an essential nutrient for some animals, but humans not only get considerable amounts in the diet, in free form and as an integral component of lecithin, but they can also synthesize it. There should be no concern about any specific intake, except perhaps during rapid growth.

Choline is an ingredient of several important tissues and substances, concerned particularly with nerve transmission and with the maintenance of cell membranes.

Richest sources: Egg yolk
Soybeans
Grains
Legumes
Peanuts
Liver

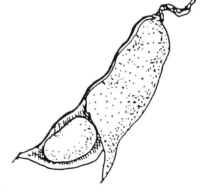

There is no established minimum requirement and there are no recognized deficiency diseases or toxicity. Choline is being added to infant formulas to bring them up to the standard of human milk. Supplements are also being tried to improve memory in the elderly and to treat alcoholic liver disease.

Average daily intake: 500 to 900 mg

Large supplemental doses of choline can cause salivation, nausea and sweating, and give the body a fishy odor.

Choline is sometimes classified as a vitamin, but this is not justified.

ARTIFICIAL FATS

We have entered the era of low-calorie and noncaloric fat substitutes. Some day they may become as commonplace as the noncaloric sweeteners that serve as sugar substitutes.

Tests on safety and palatability are being conducted by several companies and scientific groups. The following three products seem to be promising candidates.

Simplesse (NutraSweet/Monsanto) is made from milk and egg white. It has 15 percent of the calories of regular fat. Simplesse is not intended for cooking or frying, but rather for incorporation into high-fat foods such as cheese.

Olestra (Procter & Gamble) is made from table sugar (sucrose) and several oils, combined into a synthetic molecule that cannot be absorbed by the gastrointestinal tract. It might be used initially as a partial component of conventional fats used in cooking and frying, but has potential uses as a complete fat substitute.

Salatrim (Nabisco) is a fat with lowered calories, providing five calories per gram instead of the usual nine calories. The lowering of calories is brought about by incomplete absorption and utilization of the compound. The letters in Salatrim stand for "short and long chain acid triglyceride molecule." Salatrim will initially be available to food producers.

FASCINATING FACTS ABOUT FAT

- Ounce for ounce, cheddar cheese contains more cholesterol than steak, and three times as much saturated fat.
- A glass of whole milk provides more saturated fat and more cholesterol than four slices of bacon.

- Coconut oil contains 50 percent more saturated fat than butter and more than twice as much as lard.
- Cod-liver oil contains two-and-a-half times as much cholesterol as butter.
- Unsaturated fat contains just as many calories as saturated fat.
- Margarine has just as many calories as butter.
- Half a cup of gourmet ice cream contains as much saturated fat as two tablespoons of lard.
- Although tofu contains no cholesterol and very little saturated fat, it gets half its calories from fat. By comparison, skinless chicken breast gets 18 percent from fat.
- Fat-free mayonnaise makes more sense than cholesterol- free mayonnaise, since mayonnaise contains very little cholesterol to begin with. For the sake of comparison, four types of mayonnaise are listed below. Values apply to one tablespoon.

	Calories	% Fat Cals	Cholesterol
Regular mayonnaise	100	99	5 mg
Cholesterol-free	90	99	0
Miracle Whip Light	40	0	0
Kraft Free	10	0	0

- Half the fat in chicken and turkey is in the skin or right beneath it. (This is not true for cholesterol.)
- There is no evidence that eating at bedtime leads to fat deposition, or that exercise after eating prevents it. When it comes to weight changes, the determining factors in healthy individuals are caloric intake and caloric expenditure, regardless of time of day.

CHAPTER 4

Vitamins:
Some Real, Some Fanciful

The term "vitamin" comes from the Latin "vita" which means "life"; it is a fitting label.

Vitamins are complex organic compounds that must be provided in the diet to facilitate a variety of metabolic processes. The human body cannot produce these essential substances, or it produces inadequate amounts even though only very small quantities are needed.

Vitamins are classified as "fat-soluble" or "water-soluble." This is noteworthy only because fat-soluble vitamins require some fat in the diet to be absorbed. Vitamins A, D, E, and K fall into this group. The B vitamins and vitamin C, on the other hand, are water-soluble and therefore easily absorbed. By the same token, however, they are also readily excreted and a daily intake is advisable. Fat-soluble vitamins are stored in the body to some degree. Cooking, processing, and prolonged storage can cause a loss of some C and B vitamins; the fat-soluble ones are less vulnerable.

There are eight essential B vitamins: thiamin (B_1), riboflavin (B_2), niacin (B_3), pyridoxine (B_6), vitamin B_{12}, folate, biotin, and pantothenic acid. Several other substances lay claim to being B vitamins such as choline, PABA, inositol, and pangamic acid but these substances do not fulfill the criteria of vitamins.

A "balanced diet" is likely to supply sufficient amounts of vitamins, but many diets are imperfect, and in such cases vitamin supplements may be helpful. A multivitamin should be based on RDA doses with its ingredients clearly labeled. If extra amounts of one or another vitamin are desired, these should be bought separately. Experts have yet to agree on the merits of *any* vitamin supplementation.

VITAMIN A (RETINOL AND BETA-CAROTENE)

Vitamin A is essential in many processes. It promotes normal growth and bone formation, maintains good vision, produces healthy skin and mucous membranes, helps avert infection, and, as an antioxidant, may play a protective role against environmental toxins and cancer-causing agents.

Vitamin A is fat-soluble, which allows for some degree of storage (chiefly in the liver). In our diet it is derived from two different food groups. Animal products give us retinol, a ready-made vitamin A. Plants supply beta-carotene, which is then converted to retinol in the body. In a balanced diet these sources are about equally represented.

Vitamin A nomenclature can be confusing. One microgram of vitamin A is now often expressed as one RE (retinol equivalent). Microgram for microgram beta-carotene is about one-sixth as potent as retinol. Occasionally UPS units or international units (IU) are used. Each of these units equals 0.3 mcg of retinol or about 1.8 mcg of beta-carotene.

Recommended Dietary Allowances
  Men: 1,000 RE
  Women: 800 RE

Vitamin A deficiency occurs when there is general malnutrition, or with impaired fat absorption, or when the diet is specifically restricted with regard to vitamin A, such as may be seen in societies where rice is the main food source. In malnourished children vitamin A deficiency most often results from a lack of milk, eggs, and other animal protein foods rather than a low beta-carotene intake.

Deficiency leads to night blindness, dry eyes, thickened skin and recurrent, sometimes fatal, infections. In children there is impaired growth, and, ultimately, blindness. In areas of poor nutrition, the devastating effects of vitamin A deficiency can be prevented at very low cost with oral supplements or with a weekly injection.

Richest sources of retinol:
  Fish liver oils
  Liver
  Fortified dairy products
  Egg yolks
Richest sources of beta-carotene:
  Yellow vegetables (carrots, yams, pumpkins)
  Fleshy orange fruits (melons, apricots, mangoes)
  Dark green vegetables

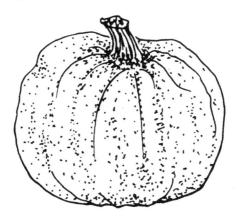

Vitamin A *toxicity* can *also* be a serious problem. Except in specific and supervised situations, retinol supplements should not exceed the daily requirement. Excessive amounts over a period of time can result in dry peeling skin, hair loss, blurred vision, bone and joint pain, headaches, irritability, abdominal pain, and liver damage. Taken during pregnancy, large doses can lead to abnormalities in the offspring. In young children, toxic amounts of retinol can actually retard growth and mental development. Excess intake *must be avoided.*

By contrast, beta-carotene supplements are well tolerated in high doses. Beta-carotene is advocated as an antioxidant; for this intended purpose amounts as high as 80,000 units are being taken with no serious side effects reported to date. When very large quantities of vegetables and fruits are eaten in the diet, the conversion to vitamin A is limited by need; the only adverse effect will be yellowing of the skin until the big doses are discontinued.

VITAMIN D
(CHOLECALCIFEROL, CALCIFEROL)

Vitamin D regulates growth and bone repair and helps to control the proper hardness of bone and teeth. It also participates in important reactions in the liver and kidneys. All these activities are closely tied to the vitamin's role in the absorption and regulation of calcium and phosphorus (phosphate).

Vitamin D is stored to some degree, chiefly in the liver. Because it is fat soluble, fat is required for its absorption.

Recommended Dietary Allowances of Cholecalciferol
   Ages 19–24: 10 mcg
   Age 25 plus: 5 mcg

Ten mcg cholecalciferol is equivalent to 400 IU of vitamin D (which is the older nomenclature).

In children, deficiency causes irritability, muscle spasms, and the retarded and defective growth pattern known as rickets. Although sunlight is the best inducer of vitamin D, rickets is not rare in tropical and subtropical climates. There can be several reasons for this: one, infants in tropical areas are often swaddled and kept indoors; two, the sun is avoided for the sake of appearance; and three, dark skin does not absorb sunlight as well as light skin. In northern countries where sunlight is scarcer, rickets occurs in regions where milk is not fortified with vitamin D.

Vitamin D deficiency in adults causes softening of bones and teeth, poor muscle tone, and impaired kidney function.

Richest sources: Sunlight effect on the skin
                Fortified dairy products and margarine
                Fortified bread and cereal products

Fish liver oil
Fish
Egg yolk

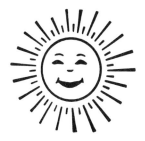

Excessive doses of vitamin D, usually in the form of supplements, can have serious consequences, particularly in children. At only five times the recommended dose (a relatively small margin), there may be permanent damage to the heart and kidneys. Lesser symptoms of overdose include weakness, thirst, loss of appetite, vomiting, and headaches.

VITAMIN E

Vitamin E comprises a group of oily substances of which alpha-tocopherol is the most active and the most available in nature.

It has long been known that this vitamin is needed by many animal species, and that serious deficiency symptoms develop when it is withheld. In human beings, deficiency is seen only with illnesses that interfere with normal fat absorption and in premature infants. When it occurs, it is characterized by neurologic dysfunction and visual problems.

Deficiencies aside, vitamin E is primarily considered an antioxidant, trapping free radicals and protecting cells and cell membranes. It does this in collaboration with other antioxidants: selenium, vitamin C, and vitamin A. Numerous claims have been made for vitamin E by proponents who believe that large amounts are valuable even when no deficiency can be demonstrated. Vitamin E is being advocated to enhance fertility (tocopherol actually means oil of fertility); to improve sexual potency; to slow down the aging process; to prevent cancer, heart attacks, and lung clots; and to treat ulcers, breast cysts, skin diseases, and poor circulation. None of these claims has been proved in a controlled setting, but many serious studies are in progress, and it is possible that the RDA will be increased in the foreseeable future.

Recommended Dietary Allowances
Men: 10 α-TE
Women: 8 α-TE

Perplexing as all the health claims are, the nomenclature, as found on food products and vitamin supplements, is even more confusing. The unit used here, α-TE, stands for alpha Tocopherol Equivalent. One α-TE is equal to the activity of 1 mg of d-α-tocopherol, also known as RRR-α-tocopherol. This is the naturally occurring form of the compound. The synthetic form is dl-α-tocopherol; it is 26 percent less active (d and l are mirror forms of a molecule, d standing for right and l for left). One mg of dl-α-tocopherols is equivalent to 1 IU, which is yet another designation. If a label uses IUs, the RDA should be 14 for men and 11 for women.

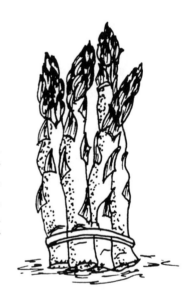

Richest sources: *Wheat germ oil*
  Other vegetable oils
  Nuts and seeds
  Green vegetables
  Egg yolk
  Butter

Large doses of vitamin E are well tolerated. People who take forty or eighty times the recommended dose seem to have no problems. Hair loss, fatigue, muscle weakness, and diarrhea have been reported with even greater amounts.

VITAMIN K

Vitamin K is a fat-soluble vitamin necessary for the normal clotting of blood. Human requirements are very small and are generally met by the average diet. A form of vitamin K is also produced by the intestine, but it is uncertain how much of that is utilized.

Recommended Dietary Allowances
  Men aged 19–24:   *70 mcg*
  Men aged 25 plus: *80 mcg*
  Women aged 19–24:   *60 mcg*
  Women aged 25 plus: *65 mcg*

Excessive bleeding ensues when there is a significant deficiency of vitamin K. Such a deficiency is most likely to occur in a newborn (whose diet is inadequate and whose intestine is not yet geared up to produce the vitamin), and in individuals with intestinal disease who are unable to eat or who are receiving antibiotics that sterilize the bowel.

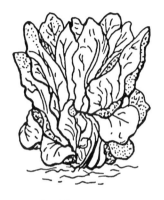

Richest sources: Green vegetables
Green tea
Soybean oil
Milk and dairy products
Liver

Toxicity occurs only when an overdose of vitamin K is given as a drug. An excess causes serious damage to red blood cells. Vitamin K is not included in multivitamin preparations, and unlike the other fat-soluble vitamins, is not stored by the body to any significant degree.

VITAMIN C (ASCORBIC ACID)

Vitamin C has many essential functions. It is involved with amino acid metabolism, hormone production, bone and tooth formation, normal growth, wound healing, and maintenance of cell membranes. It also plays a role in immune responses and allergic reactions.

Recommended Dietary Allowance: 60 mg

Increasingly vitamin C is also being viewed as an important antioxidant. For this role particularly, much larger amounts are being advocated by some scientists, with doses up to 100 times as great as the recommended allowance. Various benefits are cited, including a lessening of cold symptoms, lowering of blood cholesterol levels, improved wound healing, protection against pollutants and environmental toxins, improved adaptation to stress, and a general bolstering of the immune system. However, studies to date have not been compelling enough to persuade the medical community, so the recommended daily allowance stands.

Man is unable to produce vitamin C in the body nor can the vitamin be stored for any length of time. It must therefore be taken every day, either in the diet or by supplement. Overcooking destroys vitamin C. (Overcooking may consist of cooking too long, or cooking in too much water, or at too high a temperature.)

Richest sources: Green peppers
Citrus fruit
Cabbage varieties
Collard greens
Other green vegetables
Potatoes
Tomatoes

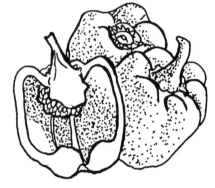

Deficiency can lead to easy bruising, bleeding gums, tissue swelling (edema), muscle and joint tenderness, increased susceptibility to infection, poor wound healing, fatigue, and ultimately scurvy, the full-blown vitamin C deficiency disease, which is manifested by anemia, loosening of teeth, hemorrhages, and finally death. The description of scurvy among British sailors 250 years ago is a medical classic and has given us the term "limey," but actually the condition was recognized some centuries earlier among explorers and seafarers deprived of fresh fruits and vegetables for prolonged periods. Today scurvy is most likely to occur in infants and young children sustained entirely on cow's milk.

Vitamin C toxicity is rarely encountered, even with very large doses, but massive amounts could interfere with the activity of anticoagulants (blood thinners) and vitamin B_{12}. Kidney stones have been blamed on vitamin C excess, but this connection has yet to be proved. The same goes for reports of fatigue, insomnia, nausea, and diarrhea.

When a high intake of vitamin C is discontinued suddenly, the body may perceive this as a deficiency. It is a type of withdrawal effect, and could be particularly serious in a newborn whose mother took large amounts during pregnancy.

THE B VITAMINS

The B vitamins are grouped together because they were originally identified as a group. They are often found in the same sorts of food, and deficiencies, when they occur, tend to involve several of them. The eight essential Bs are thiamine, riboflavin, niacin, pyridoxine, vitamin B_{12}, folate, biotin, and pantothenic acid.

THIAMINE (VITAMIN B_1)

Thiamine is required for many bodily processes such as the metabolism of carbohydrates and the normal functioning of the heart and nervous system. It is water-soluble and therefore not stored in the body to any great degree.

Recommended Dietary Allowances
   Men aged 19–50:   *1.5 mg*
   Men aged 51 plus: *1.2 mg*
   Women aged 19–50:   *1.1 mg*
   Women aged 51 plus: *1.0 mg*

Deficiency in its full-blown form leads to beriberi, a disease that affects the heart, nerves, and muscles, as well as mental functioning. Milder cases may manifest themselves in weakness, loss of appetite, constipation, pain and tingling of arms and legs, insomnia, irritability, and cardiac symptoms.

As is true for other B vitamins, thiamine deficiency rarely occurs as an isolated condition, but rather tends to be associated with other deficiencies of the B complex. This is not surprising, because many dietary sources are common to the whole group. Nevertheless, in societies that depend on white polished rice as their main staple, specific thiamine deficiency is not uncommon. Alcoholics are also at risk; thiamine deficiency can precipitate severe brain damage.

Richest sources: Whole grains
                Enriched cereals
                Lean meats, especially pork

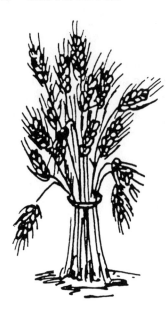

Organ meats
Nuts
Legumes

Toxicity is not a problem because excessive amounts are excreted. Allergic reactions may occur when the vitamin is given by injection.

RIBOFLAVIN (VITAMIN B₂)

Riboflavin is required for growth and metabolism, and for the maintenance of healthy skin. It also sustains the linings of the digestive tract, lungs, and blood vessels.

Recommended Dietary Allowances
    Men aged 19–50:   1.7 mg
    Men aged 51 plus: 1.4 mg
    Women aged 19–50:   1.3 mg
    Women aged 51 plus: 1.2 mg

Deficiency causes sores at the angles of the mouth, skin ailments, eye problems, and personality disorders. It occurs most frequently in alcoholics and is usually associated with other B vitamin deficiencies.

Richest sources: Milk and dairy products
            Organ meats
            Eggs
            Green vegetables
            Enriched cereals
            Bread

Toxicity is not a problem, because only limited amounts of the vitamin are absorbed.

NIACIN (NICOTINAMIDE, NIACINAMIDE, NICOTINIC ACID, VITAMIN B₃)

Niacin plays a vital role in cell metabolism and is required for the disposition of fats and carbohydrates. It also assists in the production of some hormones. Unlike most other vitamins, niacin can be synthesized by the body if the appropriate nutrients are provided (particularly tryptophan).

Niacin also differs in another way: it has functions apart from those of a vitamin. In large doses it reduces cholesterol in the blood, particularly the most undesirable fractions. Such large doses, however, can have unpleasant side effects.

Recommended Dietary Allowances
*   Men aged 19–50:   19 mg*
*   Men aged 51 plus: 15 mg*
*   Women aged 19–50:   15 mg*
*   Women aged 51 plus: 13 mg*

Deficiency is most likely to occur in alcoholics, and in populations whose chief food staple is corn (Mexico) or millet seed (India). It causes skin problems, sore tongue, loss of appetite, weakness, intestinal upsets, irritability, and depression. The full-blown form is known as pellagra and is characterized by the "three D's": diarrhea, dermatitis (rash) and dementia (mental deterioration). Outbreaks of pellagra still occur in refugee populations deprived of an adequate diet.

Niacin has been added to bread and cereal products labeled "enriched."

Richest sources: Liver and other organ meats
*   Meat*
*   Poultry and fish*
*   Peanuts and peanut*
*   butter*
*   Enriched cereals and*
*   breads*
*   Green vegetables*
*   Nuts*
*   Legumes*

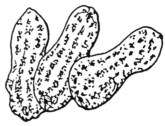

In large doses nicotinic acid (but not nicotinamide) causes flushing, itching and hives, and overactivity of the intestinal tract. In sensitive individuals it may provoke an asthmatic attack.

PYRIDOXINE (VITAMIN B$_6$)

Pyridoxine is required for the formation of red blood cells and plays an essential role in amino acid and fatty acid metabolism. It also aids in numerous other enzyme reactions. Pyridoxine works closely with other B vitamins, and particularly contributes to the functions of niacin. Pyridoxine requirements increase in high protein diets.

Recommended Dietary Allowances
Men: *2.0 mg*
Women: *1.6 mg*

Deficiency is rare except in cases of alcoholism and severe malnutrition. When it occurs, it may be manifested by nausea, weight loss, anemia, sores of the skin and mouth, and nerve damage. In infants, severe deficiency can cause seizures and mental retardation.

Richest sources: Blackstrap molasses
Liver and other organ meats
Poultry and fish
Eggs
Whole grains
Nuts
Legumes
Bananas
Avocados

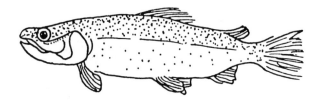

When given in supplemental doses, pyridoxine interferes with the utilization of some drugs, particularly certain medications used in epilepsy and in Parkinson's disease. Excessive doses are toxic to the nervous system, and cause numbness and tingling of the hands and feet and unsteadiness in walking. Dependency can also develop so that rapid withdrawal of substantial doses may produce deficiency symptoms which in turn may again harm the nervous system.

VITAMIN B$_{12}$ (COBALAMIN, CYANOCOBALAMIN)

Vitamin B$_{12}$ is required for all cell production. Deficiency is displayed particularly in cells that have a rapid turnover, such as red blood cells.

Recommended Dietary Allowance: 2.0 mcg

To be utilized, this vitamin requires the presence of intrinsic factor, a substance normally elaborated by the stomach. Intrinsic factor is absent in pernicious anemia and in some conditions that destroy the stomach lining. In the absence of intrinsic factor, or if there is intestinal disease, dietary B$_{12}$ cannot be utilized, and must therefore be given by injection.

Long-term vitamin B$_{12}$ deficiency causes widespread damage to the nervous system with neurologic and psychiatric symptoms. There is also anemia, burning tongue, pallor, and fatigue.

In the presence of intrinsic factor, B$_{12}$ deficiency does not occur in otherwise healthy individuals except possibly in strict vegetarians or in some elderly on a very poor diet—and then only after some months or years of deprivation.

Richest sources: Liver and other organ meats
Egg yolks
Dairy products
Meat
Fish
Fortified cereals

When there is no specific deficiency of vitamin B$_{12}$ or of intrinsic factor, shots of B$_{12}$ or of liver extract serve no useful purpose.

FOLATE (FOLIC ACID, FOLACIN)

Folic acid, one of the B vitamins, works closely with vitamin B_{12} toward normal cell production, and is particularly important during rapid growth and in pregnancy. Unlike vitamin B_{12}, folate is found in a great variety of foods, including vegetables, but it is also destroyed more easily, especially with prolonged cooking.

Even a balanced diet may not provide enough of this vitamin to women of childbearing age. Recent studies have shown that adequate folic acid intake during pregnancy prevents a certain type of birth defect. The FDA recommends that small amounts of folic acid be added to bread and cereal products, specifically flour, pasta, rice and cornmeal; and that products ought to contain folic acid if they are labeled "enriched."

Folate supplements have also been suggested for people with heart disease who are found to have high homocysteine levels. Homocysteine is an amino acid that can damage blood vessels; folate may counteract this effect.

Recommended Dietary Allowances
Men: *200 mcg*
Women aged 19 to 50: *400 mcg*
Women aged 51 plus: *180 mcg*

Deficiency causes the formation of abnormal blood cells and ultimately anemia. It may be the result of poor nutrition, alcoholism, intestinal disease which impairs folate absorption, or certain drugs that interfere with folate utilization. Unlike vitamin B_{12} deficiency, folate deficiency does not produce neurologic symptoms in adults.

When a pregnant woman is folate deficient, the birth defects in the fetus are related to the development of the nervous system. Rural China has the highest incidence of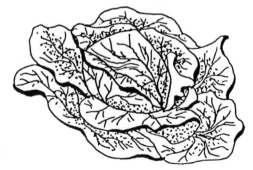

such malformations. It is said that, because the Chinese New Year is considered propitious for weddings, many babies are conceived in winter, a time when the diet lacks fresh green vegetables.

Richest sources: Fresh green vegetables
Liver and other organ meats
Egg yolks
Fortified breakfast cereals
Legumes
Bananas

Even large doses of folate are well tolerated. Nevertheless, folic acid should not be taken in doses greater than 1000 mcg, and particularly not for unspecified anemia, because the response to folic acid can mask the anemia caused by vitamin B_{12} deficiency and allow neurologic damage to proceed.

BIOTIN

Biotin, one of the B vitamins, is involved in protein, fat, and carbohydrate metabolism and may also help to maintain the texture of skin and hair.

Estimated daily requirement: 30 to 100 mcg

Deficiency is exceedingly rare because some amounts of biotin can be synthesized in the intestine. Nevertheless, it can occur with long-term biotin-deficient intravenous feeding, or with the prolonged ingestion of very large quantities of raw egg whites (20 or more raw eggs a day!). Excessive consumption of raw egg whites causes biotin deficiency

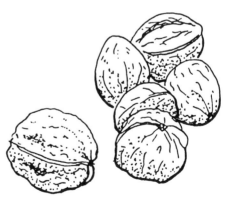

because raw egg white contains a unique substance that binds to biotin making it unavailable for its usual functions. Under these very rare and bizarre conditions, biotin deficiency causes scaling of the skin, hair loss, sore tongue, muscle pain, loss of appetite, weakness, and mental depression.

Richest sources:
  Liver and other organ meats
  Peanuts
  Walnuts
  Peanut butter
  Egg yolks
  Chocolate

Toxicity from high dosages has not been demonstrated.

PANTOTHENIC ACID (PANTOTHENATE, VITAMIN B₅)

Similar in function to several other essential B vitamins, pantothenic acid is required for the metabolism of proteins, carbohydrates, and fats; it is also necessary for the maintenance of normal skin and internal organ linings, and for the production of some hormones. The name means "obtained from everywhere" and, true to its name, this vitamin is widely available in foods.

Estimated daily requirement: 4–7 mg

Deficiency has not been clearly demonstrated in man, although there have been reports of burning feet, headache, fatigue, and depression when a deficiency was deliberately induced. Even very poor diets seem to satisfy the minimum requirement.

Richest sources: Liver and other
              organ meats
              Egg yolk
              Mushrooms
              Whole grains
              Enriched cereals
              Peanuts

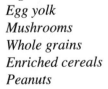

Toxicity is not known. Large doses have been taken without ill effect.

MYO-INOSITOL AND PHYTIC ACID

There are several inositols. The one usually considered in human nutrition is myo-inositol. It is present in various forms in plants and animals. In some plants, especially in cereal grains, it exists in the form of phytic acid.

Extensive animal studies have been done, but the significance of myo-inositol for humans has not been fully elucidated. It appears to play a role in fat metabolism and is reported to reduce the accumulation of cholesterol and triglycerides. It may also contribute to normal nerve conduction. Whatever its nutrient function, however, myo-inositol does not qualify as a vitamin, even though it is sometimes grouped with the B complex. Structurally it is related to glucose.

Adequate quantities are apparently produced by the body, especially in the intestine, so that it is difficult to establish a minimum need or a deficiency syndrome. The average daily intake is about 1 gm, mostly from plant foods. Inositol is often added to infant formulas, because human milk contains about three times as much as cow's milk. No deleterious effects have been reported from large supplemental doses of inositol.

Excessive amounts of phytic acid, however, eaten in the form of cereal grains and grain products, may tie up some minerals, especially calcium, iron, and zinc, and interfere with their absorption. It is interesting that zinc deficiency was first described in the Near East in men on high-phytate cereal grain diets.

PABA, PANGAMIC ACID, AND OTHER NONVITAMINS

This group is the darling of self-styled nutrition mavens and health food promoters.

PABA (para-aminobenzoic acid) is often grouped with the B vitamins ("B_x"), but by prevailing criteria it is not a vitamin in man. It is widely distributed in nature and also produced in the intestine. There is no established requirement and no known deficiency state or toxicity. PABA is used on the skin as a sunscreen agent. Claims that it prevents hair loss and graying of hair are not justified.

Pangamic acid is not a vitamin either. It is a substance of variable composition and dubious value, touted by some as a B vitamin ("B$_{15}$") and advocated to counteract aging, heart disease, and liver damage. "Pan" means "all" and "gam" means "seed"; pangamic acid is indeed derived from seeds and from the large pits of fleshy fruits. There is no known requirement or deficiency syndrome. Depending on the specific ingredients, pangamic acid supplements may not be safe.

Laetrile and **amygdalin** are derived from fruit kernels and from almonds. (Amygdalin means almond.) Once called vitamin B$_{17}$ and hailed as a cancer cure, this pair of related substances has been found ineffective, and can be toxic because the preparations contain a significant amount of cyanide.

"Vitamin P" consists of citrin, hesperidin, rutin, quercetin, and other flavonoids, a group of substances obtained from plants, especially citrus fruits. Claims on their behalf are numerous; these substances are said to prevent easy bruising and strokes, increase the resistance to allergies and colds, and help to reduce high blood pressure and elevated blood cholesterol. In controlled studies the claims have not been borne out. Quercetin supplements probably are not safe.

"Vitamin U" is yet another pseudovitamin, this one extracted from cabbage leaves. It has been promoted for the treatment of peptic ulcers.

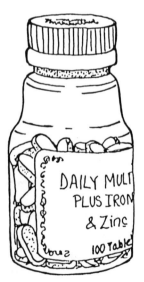

FASCINATING FACTS ABOUT VITAMINS

- The term *vitamin* comes from the Latin vita (life) and denotes a substance essential for life. The word is often used loosely, however, and more than a few compounds are sold as vitamins even though there is no proven dietary need for them and no deficiency syndrome has been demonstrated.

- The total combined weight of all eight essential B vitamins is about 31 mg per day. That means that one ounce would satisfy the needs of nine hundred people.
- Surplus vitamins do not increase energy or enhance athletic performance.
- It has never been shown that a natural vitamin is superior to a synthetic one, except in the case of vitamin E (d-α tocopherol is superior to the dl-α form.)
- Vitamins do not contribute any calories.

CHAPTER 5

Minerals: Some Essential, Some Deadly

Minerals are essential nutrients. Like vitamins, they are required in the diet for normal growth and functioning. Unlike vitamins, they are inorganic substances; that is, they are simple chemical elements rather than complex carbon compounds. And, unlike vitamins, they are actually incorporated into cells and tissues.

Some minerals are present in the body in relatively large amounts; these are sodium, potassium, calcium, magnesium, chlorine (as chloride), phosphorus (as phosphate), and sulfur.

Other minerals are required in much smaller quantities; these are the trace elements, also known as trace minerals or microminerals. This group includes iron, manganese, zinc, copper, fluorine (as fluoride), iodine, selenium, chromium, cobalt, and molybdenum. All perform important functions. There are others yet whose role and significance are still being studied; among them are boron, nickel, tin, silicon, and vanadium.

With good health, the mineral levels in the blood are amazingly constant. When blood levels threaten to drop, the body will deplete its own stores in an attempt to maintain a steady state, such as by taking calcium out of bones. Small amounts of excess can also be handled. These mechanisms are delicate and complex however, and can break down if the system is upset. Certain drugs, such as diuretics (water pills), can cause selective losses of some minerals, as can prolonged vomiting and diarrhea.

The delicate balance can also be upset when excessive doses of a mineral are taken as supplements. This can start a cascade of abnormalities affecting one or more of the other minerals and their function.

SODIUM

Sodium chloride is the combination of sodium and chlorine known to all of us as table salt. Sodium makes up 39 percent of the salt molecule, chlorine the rest.

Salt has been prized throughout the ages. In certain times and places it was considered more valuable than gold. The word "salary" is an anglicized version of "salt money" because salt was used as part payment in ancient Greece and Rome.

Salt has also left its mark in many superstitions: if you spill it, throw salt over your left shoulder, to prevent bad luck. It's bad luck to put salt on another person's plate ("help me to salt, help me to sorrow"). Give a new baby a gift of salt for good luck. (This may be a relic of Roman times, when Salus, the goddess of health, ordained that newborns have a little salt placed on their tongues right after birth.) Salt was thrown on altar fires and on the floor of a new household. Oaths were often taken on salt. (I hope the reader takes all this with a grain of salt.)

Salt is an essential ingredient of the human diet, but hardly in the quantities that we consume. As long as four thousand years ago, Chinese medical writings warn against a high salt intake. Except under unusual conditions, we get an adequate amount of salt from a balanced diet without ever using a salt shaker. Even with increased salt loss, such as occurs with profuse sweating, it is generally more important to replace the water than the salt.

Estimated daily requirement of sodium: 500 mg

This amount translates to about ¼ of a teaspoon of salt a day, including all the salt naturally present in food or added during processing. As can be seen from the chart below, a glass of tomato juice or a half cup of cottage cheese will just about meet the need. The average intake in the United States is 4,000 — 5,000 mg/day, almost ten times the amount needed; among some ethnic groups in the United States it is twice that number.

In the past several decades a lot of research has gone into studying the possible adverse effects of sodium. In predisposed individuals, excessive salt intake seems to promote and aggravate high blood pressure. A cause-and-effect relationship, however, has not been scientifically demonstrated. It is clear that the increase in blood pressure seen with advancing age is more marked in modern societies in which salt consumption is high. Unfortunately we don't know which specific individuals are susceptible to high sodium intake, but the following groups should be careful: people with high blood pressure, African Americans, the elderly, and the obese.

A high salt intake also decreases calcium retention because it increases calcium loss in the urine. People with low calcium levels should avoid too much salt in their diet.

Our taste for salt is acquired. Since excessive amounts could be harmful, it makes sense not to introduce saltiness to infants and young children in the mistaken belief that it will make food more appealing; it actually only creates an unhealthful eating pattern. We should also realize that a taste that is learned can also be unlearned regardless of one's age.

A food or drug that has the word "sodium" or "soda" in its name contains salt in one form or another. A label reading "reduced sodium" means that the item contains at least 25 percent less salt than the standard product. "Low sodium" indicates 140 mg or less per serving (but a serving may be smaller than expected). "Very low sodium" means 35 mg or less, and "sodium free" means less than 5 mg of sodium per serving.

Salt substitutes usually are compounds that replace the sodium with potassium to produce a potassium salt. They are not risk-free, especially when taken with some medications or when kidney function is impaired; however, they do provide a salty taste.

Three-quarters of the salt we eat is part of processed food, rather than added in cooking or at the table. Among the saltiest foods are those that are pickled, canned, smoked or cured. (Canned soup may be "good food," but it often contains lots of salt.) Salty taste is definitely not a reliable indicator of the actual salt content. Ounce for ounce, for example, some dry cereals contain more salt than potato chips.

The following list gives some examples of sodium content:

	Sodium (mg)
FLAVORINGS	
Table salt, 1 tsp.	2,300
Soy sauce, 1 tbs.	1,030
Catsup, 1 tbs.	156
Mustard, 1 tbs.	190
Italian salad dressing, 1 tbs.	315
GRAIN PRODUCTS	
Pepperidge Farm white bread, 1 slice	123
Wonder bread, white, 1 slice	175
Saltine crackers, 3 pieces	120
Corn flakes, 1 oz	320
Cheerios, 1 oz	290
Shredded or puffed wheat, puffed rice or wheat	0
SNACKS	
Potato chips, 1 oz	210
Salted peanuts, 1 oz	138
Pretzels, 1 oz	450
LUNCH FOODS	
Bologna, 1 oz slice	285
Boiled ham, 1 oz slice	375
Dry salami, 1 oz	633
Pork sausage, 1 link, 2 oz	800
Frankfurter, 2 oz	650
Tuna, canned in oil or water, 6½ oz can	910
American cheese, 1 oz slice	390
Cottage cheese, ½ cup	460
FAST FOOD	
McDonald's Big Mac	1,010
Burger King Whopper	990
CANNED SOUPS	
Black bean soup, 1 cup	1,200
Chicken noodle soup, 1 cup	1,100
Manhattan clam chowder, 1 cup	1,600
Tomato soup, 1 cup	875
BEVERAGES	
Club soda, 1 cup	55
Orange juice, 1 cup	2
Tomato juice, 1 cup	486
MISCELLANEOUS	
Dill pickle	900
Sauerkraut, ½ cup	777

POTASSIUM

Potassium is one of the major minerals in the body. It is found chiefly *within* cells rather than in body fluids. Along with the other electrolytes, sodium and chloride, potassium helps regulate fluid balance in the body. It is also important in the transmission of nerve impulses, for the control of heart rhythm, and for the smooth functioning of muscles.

Estimated daily requirement: 2,000 mg

Potassium is widely available in food, particularly unprocessed food, and deficiency does not occur under ordinary conditions. Prolonged vomiting or diarrhea, however, results in potassium loss. In a similar vein some diuretics (water pills), laxatives, and heart medications increase the need for potassium, and supplements may be required; these should be taken only under a physician's supervision.

Potassium deficiency is serious. It leads to muscle weakness, lethargy, and may cause heart rhythm disturbances.

Potassium is abundant in most vegetables, fruits, meats, and fish. For quick potassium restoration, bananas, orange juice, and tomato juice are good choices. Other rich sources are dried fruits, melons, nuts, and peanut butter. Most salt substitutes also contain a high concentration of potassium.

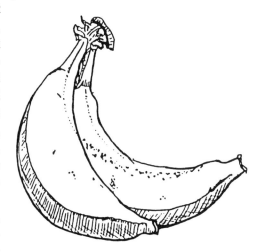

As with many nutrients, the human body is amazingly adept at utilizing the amount of potassium that it needs and then excreting the rest as long as the potassium comes from food sources. In this way the mineral is absorbed at an appropriate pace, transferred into cells, and never allowed to exceed a safe level in the circulation. (This can be said only for healthy individuals; in some conditions, particularly kidney disease, potassium intake may have to be limited.)

When formulated as a medication, potassium is a potent drug that must be monitored with care. Potassium excess has serious consequences. Irregular heart rhythms and abnormal heart activity are the most ominous toxic effects and require emergency treatment.

CHLORIDE

Chloride is the combining form of the element chlorine. As a component of salt (sodium chloride), it occurs naturally in numerous foods and is also added to many of the foods we eat. Despite their close association, the requirements and concentrations of sodium and chloride differ, and the two elements function independently.

Chloride plays an important role in maintaining the delicate acid-base and fluid balance in the body. It is also a major ingredient of gastric acid needed for digestion in the stomach.

Estimated daily requirement: 750 mg

Deficiency does not occur with any kind of reasonable diet, although prolonged vomiting or sweating may lead to depletion. Just as with sodium, most of our supply comes from processed food and the rest from the salt shaker.

CALCIUM

Of all the major minerals, calcium is the most plentiful in the human body. Ninety-nine percent of it is found in bones. During childhood, when bones and teeth are being formed, an adequate intake is particularly important. The need never stops, however, because we constantly excrete calcium and therefore must replenish it. To complicate things further, calcium is not always absorbed and utilized properly, even when adequate amounts or supplements are ingested. This is especially true as people get older. Other measures may then have to be taken to promote calcium utilization and prevent excessive calcium loss and thinning of bones. A preventive regime is best started in early middle age; any such program should be under medical supervision.

In addition to its role in bone and tooth formation, calcium is necessary for normal blood clotting, nerve and muscle function, and regulation of heart rhythm. Recent studies suggest that adequate calcium intake also plays a role in preventing high blood pressure and possibly even cancer.

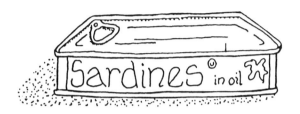

Recommended Dietary Allowances
Ages 19–24:   1,200 mg
Ages 25 plus: 800 mg

Deficiency may be due to inadequate intake, but other factors are more likely to be responsible. These include hormone imbalance (e.g. menopause), vitamin D deficiency, metabolic disturbances, and conditions that interfere with intestinal absorption. The symptoms and signs of low calcium levels in the blood are often tied to the basic cause. For example, low calcium is usually found in cases of rickets, but the primary cause in that instance is a vitamin D deficiency.

In the absence of serious disease, the body attempts to maintain a normal calcium level in the blood, even at the expense of drawing it out of the bones. If this mechanism proves inadequate, blood calcium levels drop and there may be muscle spasms, cramps, neurologic disturbances, and mental changes.

Richest sources: Milk and milk products
Sardines and other canned fish
Oysters
Green vegetables
Bean curd

Inordinate amounts of calcium in the diet can interfere with the absorption of other minerals and also cause constipation. Calcium toxicity, however, is rare because under normal conditions the body readily deals with this excess. More commonly, high calcium levels in the blood are due to other causes (just as deficiency is usually not a matter of intake alone). These causes may be hormonal or related to various disease states. Elevated calcium levels can cause abdominal upsets, weakness, and changes in behavior. Ultimately the kidneys will be damaged.

PHOSPHORUS

Phosphorus is involved in numerous activities. It is not only essential, but may in fact have more different functions than any other mineral in the body! It is required for all energy production and metabolic reactions. Phosphorus is a component of every body tissue, but eighty percent of it is found in the bones and teeth.

Recommended Dietary Allowances
   Ages 19–24:   1,200 mg
   Ages 25 plus: 800 mg

Deficiency is very rare because phosphorus is widely available, particularly in protein-rich food. It may occur, however, with excessive use of magnesium-aluminum antacids. Deficiency causes weakness and thinning of bone.

Richest sources: Eggs
               Milk and dairy products
               Meat
               Poultry
               Fish
               Whole grains
               Nuts
               Legumes

Phosphorus excess can lead to calcium loss.

MAGNESIUM

Magnesium is found chiefly in bone, but is present in all body tissues. It is essential in bone and tooth formation and for the normal functioning of nerves and muscles. Magnesium is also a component of many enzymes.

Recommended Dietary Allowances
Men: 350 mg
Women: 280 mg.

Deficiency is not uncommon. It may develop in people with poor dietary habits, heavy alcohol intake, poorly controlled diabetes, kidney disease, intestinal malabsorption, and use of phosphate drugs. Diuretics (water pills) and prolonged intravenous feeding may also reduce magnesium.

Deficiency can lead to weakness, twitching and trembling, muscle cramps (tetany), erratic behavior, and irregular heartbeat. In pregnancy, magnesium deficiency can contribute to high blood pressure.

Richest sources: Legumes
*   Green vegetables*
*   Nuts*
*   Whole grains*
*   Chocolate and cocoa*
*   Seafood*

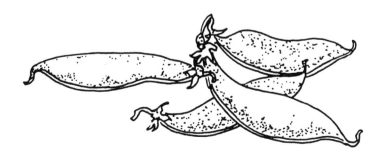

Magnesium levels may rise in some disease states, and also with the abuse of magnesium-type antacids. Excess leads to nausea, vomiting, diarrhea, and a drop in blood pressure. Ultimately respiratory failure may ensue. People with poor kidney function are especially at risk.

SULFUR

Sulfur is one of the major essential minerals, notably as a component of several amino acids, hormones, vitamins, and enzymes. It is found in all tissues, with the greatest concentration in bone, hair, and nails.

A daily requirement for sulfur has not been established.

Richest sources: Cheese
Eggs
Milk
Meat
Nuts
Legumes

A diet even barely adequate in protein will supply sufficient sulfur. Deficiency symptoms have not been described, and neither has toxicity from excessive amounts in the diet.

ESSENTIAL TRACE MINERALS

These elements, though essential, are required in very small amounts. The total substance of all the trace minerals in the human body would fit into a thimble. The essential trace elements are iron, zinc, copper, manganese, iodine, fluoride, selenium, molybdenum, chromium, and possibly cobalt.

IRON

Iron is one of the trace elements. It is found chiefly in the blood as a component of hemoglobin, and is required for the transportation of oxygen to all tissues. The bone marrow, liver, and spleen also contain substantial amounts of iron.

Recommended Dietary Allowances
Men: *10 mg*
Women aged 19–50:   *15 mg*
Women aged 51 plus: 10 mg

The human body retains iron well. It has been said that unless one is losing blood, one gets enough iron by walking by a rusty pole now and then. That is almost true. Extra needs do arise when there is blood loss, or when a greater requirement is imposed by rapid growth, pregnancy, or lactation. Despite an otherwise adequate diet, women of menstruating age often don't get enough iron if their total caloric intake is modest or if they eat no animal proteins.

Richest sources: Liver
                              Meat
                              Egg yolks
                              Dried fruits
                              Fortified cereals
                              Blackstrap molasses

Deficiency leads to anemia (thin blood), eventually manifested by pallor, fatigue, and decreased resistance to infection. There may be difficulty in swallowing. Nails may become malformed.

Vitamin C enhances iron utilization and iron cookware adds a certain amount of iron to food.

On the down side, excessive iron supplementation interferes with the absorption of zinc. In infants it can cause copper depletion. Large overdoses may be fatal in children. Adult-size supplements (which often look like candy) must be kept out of their reach.

High iron levels in the body, sometimes seen in men and postmenopausal women, have been reported to increase the risk of heart attack and intestinal polyps. One way to get rid of iron overload is by periodic bloodletting or blood donation. Medication is also available and is applied in a process known as chelation.

ZINC

Zinc is an essential component of enzymes, bones, teeth, blood cells, testes, and several other organs. Zinc also plays a role in normal growth and sexual maturation, and is important for the healthy functioning of the immune system.

Recommended Dietary Allowances
  Men: 15 mg
  Women: 12 mg

Deficiency may cause loss of taste, poor appetite, and fatigue. It can interfere with normal wound healing, physical growth, and sexual maturation.

Richest sources: Oysters
                Fish and shellfish
                Organ meats
                Meat
                Egg yolks

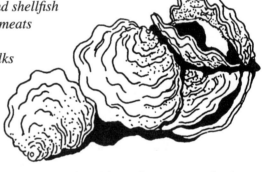

High milk consumption and high-dose iron supplementation in children can result in poor zinc absorption. Large amounts of plant protein, such as that found in soybeans, may also interfere. Zinc reserves in the body are small, and mild or marginal zinc deficiency is not rare, particularly in people who avoid animal products or who eat a lot of processed foods. (Processing often removes zinc.)

Low zinc levels have been reported in certain diseases, particularly rheumatoid arthritis, but a true deficiency has not been demonstrated nor is there any proven cause-and-effect relationship. Studies are also in progress to evaluate zinc supplementation for the prevention of visual loss in the elderly.

On the other hand, too much zinc is not harmless. It interferes with the availability of copper and iron and may thus cause anemia. It also changes the lipid profile unfavorably and may produce gastrointestinal side effects such as vomiting and diarrhea. The immune system can possibly be interfered with by too much as well as by too little zinc.

COPPER

Copper is found chiefly in bone, muscle, liver, and blood. It is required by the red blood cell for the proper utilization of iron in the production of hemoglobin. Copper also assists in amino acid metabolism and in enzyme formation.

Estimated daily requirement: 1.5–3.0 mg

Most people get adequate amounts of copper in their daily diet. Low copper levels are associated with protein malnutrition.

An inadequate copper intake may lead to anemia (thin blood) and elevation of cholesterol. Children born with a defect in copper absorption suffer from poor bone formation and retarded growth unless the condition is recognized and treated.

Richest sources: Organ meats
Shellfish
Lean meats
Legumes
Nuts

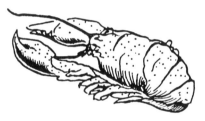

Interference with copper utilization can be brought about by large supplemental doses of zinc or megadoses of vitamin C. Inordinate copper intake is well tolerated and symptoms of toxicity are very rare; abdominal symptoms, muscle pain, and ultimately liver damage could result from prolonged excess intake of copper.

MANGANESE

Manganese is an essential component of enzymes and plays a role in nerve function and in reproduction. It is also necessary for normal bone and tendon structure.

Estimated daily requirement: 2.0–5.0 mg

Manganese is widely distributed in plant foods.

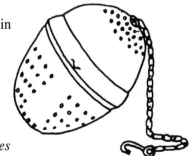

Richest sources: Whole grains
Cereal products
Peanut butter
Tea
Fruits and vegetables

A deficiency state has not been substantiated, but some research has suggested that inadequate manganese may play a role in osteoporosis. Manganese toxicity does not occur with oral intake even when very large amounts are eaten. Prolonged inhalation of manganese dust or fumes, however, can damage the nervous system, causing gait disturbances, tremors, and slurred speech.

IODINE

Iodine is one of the essential trace elements. It is readily available in areas near the ocean where it is found in the water and soil, but the natural supply may be inadequate in inland areas. As a significant component of thyroid hormone, iodine is necessary for normal thyroid activity, which controls the body's metabolism.

Recommended Dietary Allowance: 150 mcg

Deficiency of iodine causes hypothyroidism (depressed thyroid function), which results in sluggish metabolism, fatigue, and cold intolerance. Chronic lack of iodine can produce goiter.

Women who are severely deficient during pregnancy may give birth to a specific type of mentally retarded child. Not too long ago this condition, known as cretinism, was common in mountainous villages far from the sea and its bounty. Until the introduction of iodized salt, areas in Switzerland and northern Pakistan, for instance, had an inordinate number of children born with this specific type of defective growth and brain development.

Richest sources: Iodized salt
Saltwater fish
Shellfish
Dairy products

Eggs, meats, and vegetables vary widely with regard to iodine content, depending on the iodine content of the soil. It is therefore recommended that people in inland areas use iodized salt. Incidentally, the iodine in milk comes mainly from the iodine disinfectants used on dairy farms!

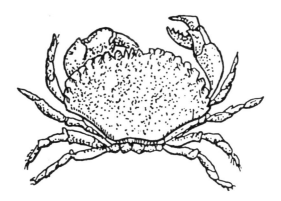

Paradoxically, high doses of iodine also suppress the thyroid, and this characteristic has been used to treat overactive thyroid glands. Goiters have actually been reported in areas where iodine-rich sea weed is a major food staple. On the whole, the body adapts well to a broad range of iodine intake, and symptoms of deficiency or excess are now rarely seen in western society.

FLUORIDE

Fluoride is the combining form of fluorine, one of the trace elements. There is some controversy about calling fluoride essential, but without much doubt it is beneficial. It contributes to firm bone structure, and is a component of tooth enamel, giving it strength and providing resistance to cavities.

Fluoride is found in almost all food and water, but not necessarily in meaningful amounts.

Estimated daily requirement: 1.5–4.0 mg

Deficiency contributes to tooth decay. In children it can also compromise the strength of bones, and in the elderly it may promote bone loss (osteoporosis).

Richest sources:
Water containing adequate fluoride
Fish, especially small fish eaten with bones
Tea

For some time now there has been a heated debate about the advisability of adding fluoride to the water supply in fluoride-poor areas. Objections are based on an aversion to forced medication, and also on the fear of toxicity. Persistent and excessive intake of fluoride can indeed cause mottling and pitting of teeth in children (fluorosis), and massive overexposure leads to kidney damage and to undue thickening and growth of bone.

In recommended doses, however, fluoridation is accepted by most scientists and health care providers as an important public health measure. One part per million (0.0001%) is the recommended amount in the water supply. It has been shown that the incidence of caries (cavities, tooth decay) is reduced significantly by fluoridation. Baby teeth also benefit from fluoride treatments by the dentist. Fluoride toothpaste and mouthwash may be helpful as well.

SELENIUM

Selenium is one of the essential trace elements. In animals it works closely alongside vitamin E as an antioxidant, and as such protects against assaults attributed to free radicals. Human data for the salutary effects are not as compelling as animal data and are still being examined.

Recommended Dietary Allowances
Men: 70 mcg
Women: 55 mcg

Drinking water in selenium-poor areas contains less than 1 mcg of selenium per quart. In selenium-rich areas there is up to 300 times as much.

Infants in selenium-poor areas, particularly in some parts of China, have a high incidence of a specific type of heart disease. This can be prevented with selenium supplementation. The only deficiency symptoms reported in adults are muscle pain and weakness after long-term intravenous feeding; this seems to respond to selenium administration.

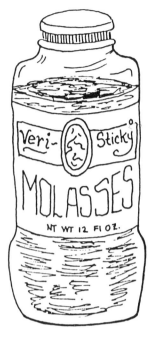

Richest sources: Organ meats
Molasses
Grains grown in selenium
rich soil
Fish and shellfish

When selenium intake is excessive over a prolonged period or with occupational exposure, toxic effects may be seen. These include hair loss, nail deformities, skin eruptions, nervousness, nausea, and offensive body odor.

MOLYBDENUM

Molybdenum is one of the trace elements considered essential because it is part of an important enzyme system. It facilitates copper and iron metabolism.

Estimated daily requirement: 75–250 mcg

Deficiency has not been described except possibly in patients who receive nothing but intravenous feedings for a prolonged period. In such a situation it is difficult to sort out what symptoms are caused by what deficiency, but apparently molybdenum supplementation alleviates some of them.

Richest sources: Grains
Grain products
Legumes
Milk

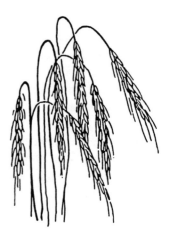

Excessive amounts of molybdenum reduce copper levels and interfere with its function. Very large doses can cause swelling of joints similar to gout.

CHROMIUM

Chromium is one of the essential trace elements. It helps maintain normal blood sugar levels and may play a role in cholesterol metabolism.

Estimated daily requirement: 50–200 mcg

Deficiency is difficult to demonstrate, but it has been shown that diabetics on inadequate intakes improve their handling of sugar when chromium supplements are given. Patients on prolonged intravenous feedings, as well as the elderly, could also be subject to deficiency and be impaired with regard to blood sugar and fat metabolism.

Richest sources: Liver
Clams
Peanuts and peanut butter
Grains and grain products
Corn oil
Some beers and wines
American cheese

No toxicity has been reported from eating large amounts of chromium-rich foods. Industrial exposure, which is hazardous, involves chromium salts and acids, compounds not found in food.

COBALT

Cobalt has no known independent function, but is a necessary constituent of vitamin B_{12}. In vegetarians who depend on the small amounts of B_{12} produced in the intestine, cobalt intake could be essential.

Estimated daily requirement: less than 1 mcg
Richest sources: Fish
Peanut butter
Organ meats

No independent deficiency symptoms have been described. Toxicity occurs only with huge doses (10,000 times the estimated need), and affects red blood cell formation and thyroid function.

TRACE ELEMENTS
NOT PROVEN ESSENTIAL

BORON

Although not yet included in the list of essential trace elements, boron may play an important role in bone metabolism and could soon be acknowledged as one of the many necessary ingredients of a healthy diet. It appears to offer protection from osteoporosis either by sparing calcium or by enhancing hormone activity when hormone levels are low thereby promoting calcium utilization. The richest sources are fruits, cabbage, nuts, and legumes. Large doses of boron are toxic to the kidneys and can be fatal. (Boron is used to kill cockroaches—a testimonial to its toxicity.)

TIN

Tin is an element not known to be required by humans, but apparently needed by some animal species for normal growth. The richest sources are cereal products (bread, crackers, pasta).

Prolonged storage of food in old-fashioned tin-alloy cans may allow some amount of tin to leach into the canned food product. If the amount is large, it can interfere with the absorption of zinc.

SILICON

The need for silicon in human nutrition has not been proved, but in some animal species it is required for orderly development of bones and connective tissue and also for maintenance of normal brain composition. High-fiber plants are the richest source.

Toxic effects are conceivable if trisilicate antacids are taken steadily over many years. More hazardous is the long-term inhalation of silica dust which has been shown to increase the risk of silicosis, a serious and potentially fatal lung disease, commonly found in miners and sand blasters.

NICKEL

Nickel may play a role in cell and cell membrane structure. Several animal species require nickel for normal growth and blood cell formation, but no dietary need has been demonstrated in man. The richest sources are oysters, grain products, legumes, cocoa, and black pepper.

VANADIUM

Vanadium is required by some animals for normal thyroid function and perhaps growth and reproduction, but it has not been proved essential in human nutrition. It is found in minute amounts in shellfish, fish, and many other foods.

TOXIC ELEMENTS

Toxic elements, many of them "heavy metals," have no proven nutritional value in man, although lead, arsenic, and cadmium, in tiny amounts, are essential in some animals. In any significant quantity they are poisonous to humans, each in a different way. Ingestion, as well as inhalation, should be avoided.

LEAD

Lead is a serious health hazard, even when health effects are not obvious or acute. Until recently, the chief source of poisoning was probably lead-based paint, eaten in the form of paint chips and peelings from the walls of old buildings, or from painted cribs and other furniture. Old crayons also contain lead. (The new ones are lead-free.)

Drinking water is now receiving some of the attention it deserves with regard to lead content. Lead contamination may come from the water source itself or from pipes made of lead or soldered with lead. Five parts per billion is considered the maximum acceptable lead level in drinking water; the level is significantly higher in many places. Some historians have said that the Roman empire fell because lead poisoning from lead water pipes was so prevalent. This is not likely, however, because the Romans were well aware of the hazards of lead plumbing.

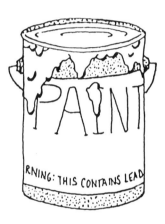

There are several more insidious sources of toxic lead: vegetables grown in soil contaminated by the remains of previous buildings; soil itself, if it is eaten in the form of clay or putty (a practice not uncommon in some areas); the sand in sand boxes; old china, particularly if the glaze has been worn away by time or dishwasher detergent; and food from very old tin cans that were soldered with lead.

Lead inhalation is also hazardous. This includes persistent exposure to leaded gasoline or the lead dust generated in many industries. Lead emissions from Greek and Roman times can still be detected in some European lake sediments after some 2,500 years! (Among the ancients, lead was a by-product of silver smelting.)

The effects of lead poisoning are usually gradual and cumulative. Lead is particularly dangerous to infants and young children, and also to pregnant women because lead is transferred to the fetus. In children, it causes mental retardation and delayed physical development. Other toxic manifestations, which can occur in adults too, are loss of appetite, anemia, irritability, weakness, high blood pressure, hearing loss, and kidney damage. Some of these effects are irreversible.

Babies should be screened for lead at one and two years of age. Thereafter blood tests should be repeated, along with a little detective work, when there is any suspicion of lead contamination. This applies particularly to the water supply. If in doubt, check it out! Most local health departments will lend assistance when the health of children is threatened. A list of public and private testing organizations is available from the Environmental Protection Agency.

MERCURY

Mercurial waste materials and fungicides may contaminate fish and agricultural products. The source of the mercury is not always clear; it may be the result of direct industrial pollution, but it may also come from emissions or dumping some distance away.

Chronic poisoning results in metallic taste, loss of appetite, anemia, kidney damage, irritability, visual problems, tremors, spasticity, mental aberrations, and, in children, mental retardation.

Mercury contained in dental fillings (amalgam) has not been shown to pose a health hazard in humans. Small amounts of mercury apparently do escape from such fillings and may be deposited in body organs. The amounts are evidently too small to result in demonstrable disease, but suspicions have been raised over the years that they can cause antibiotic resistance and other problems. More investigations may be forthcoming.

ARSENIC

Tiny quantities of arsenic are required by some animal species, and trace amounts may someday prove to be essential in the human diet.

Before the advent of antibiotics, arsenic was used in the treatment of some serious diseases, including syphilis and tuberculosis. Chronic poisoning from small doses in various medications and nostrums was not rare. Nowadays toxic effects may result from contamination by herbicides and fertilizers. Symptoms include diarrhea, garlic odor of breath and sweat, darkening of the skin (especially eyelids), disturbed sensations, loss of appetite, and weakness; ultimately there is liver and kidney failure.

Arsenic is tasteless and has been a favorite with poisoners through the ages.

CADMIUM

The use of cadmium in industry has increased over the past decades, and with this increase some cadmium has entered the food chain through contamination of water and soil. When ingested by grazing animals, cadmium is concentrated in the liver and kidneys. The organ meats of deer and moose may therefore be toxic to man and should not be eaten.

Smokers can absorb cadmium from cigarette smoke. Paint and galvanized pipes have also been impugned. Although the amounts that are absorbed are usually small, cadmium settles in the tissues and over the years can damage the kidneys and other organs. It has been suggested that cadmium exposure also contributes to hypertension.

ALUMINUM

Although often accused, aluminum utensils and cookware have never been shown to cause any damage. The debate continues, however, concerning other aluminum sources, water in particular. Abnormal aluminum deposits are found in the brains of patients with Alzheimer's disease, which has caused some people to seek a relationship between high aluminum levels in the local water supply and the incidence of this disease. Aluminum antacids are also under suspicion. There is no proof of any of this.

Inhalation of aluminum fumes and particles is another matter. Workers in aluminum smelting plants may develop neurologic problems such as loss of balance, impaired memory, and incoordination.

FASCINATING FACTS ABOUT MINERALS

- Sea water contains 3½ percent salt, or almost half a tablespoon of salt per 8 ounce glass—not as much as soy sauce, but more than almost any other food item. Even fish can't drink sea water. They either process it or obtain the necessary water from the food they eat, be it animal or vegetable.
- Even unbalanced diets are likely to supply the essential minerals in adequate amounts with several exceptions. One such mineral is iodine; in deficient areas this must be remedied with iodized salt. Another is iron, frequently deficient in premenopausal women. A third is calcium, particularly in the elderly whose diet has been calcium deficient for some years and who are not receiving hormone replacement.
- Three minerals, sodium, potassium, and chloride, comprise the major electrolytes; that means that, among other tasks, it is largely their responsibility to maintain the acid-alkali and water balance in the blood. The balance is very critical and must be precise. Even small shifts can cause major problems; large shifts are life-threatening.

CHAPTER 6

The Stuff We Eat

We have long suspected that a good diet is a keystone to health, vigor, and longevity. Defining a good diet is a bit more difficult and our concepts continue to change. Some national and ethnic groups have dietary habits that differ from what we consider prudent, and yet they seem none the worse for it.

Quite obviously many factors are at play. Man is a complex organism, affected by a myriad of variables of which diet is but one, albeit an important one. Over the past decades, nutrition experts have gathered information from many sources including population studies, clinical trials, and animal research. It behooves us to look at their findings.

Heart disease is of particular interest to Americans because the mortality rate from heart attacks is high in the U.S. The French who consume large quantities of saturated fat and cholesterol have a lower incidence of cardiac deaths; in fact they have the second lowest rate in Europe. Several questions come to mind. Since it may take decades for dietary changes to show their effect on population trends, can we assume that current statistics are a reflection of how Americans ate twenty years ago, and can we assume that outcomes will improve as people become more nutrition conscious? Are the favorable heart attack data from France and the Mediterranean, from China and Japan the result of their prior dietary habits and life styles? And will the picture change if these groups eat more fast foods and give up conventional patterns of living? One final question: are reporting methods the same in the United States and other countries? American physicians may be ascribing unexplained deaths to heart attacks or some sort of cardiac event more often than other countries, where such deaths are perhaps attributed to "natural" or "unknown" causes; this would then skew the statistics. With these caveats in mind, let us look at some specifics.

The French have posed the greatest puzzle, sometimes referred to as "the French paradox." They have far fewer heart attacks and live slightly longer than Americans, despite the fact that their diet could be considered "flawed" by current nutritional standards. The tempting explanation has been that the French drink red wine. Some preliminary reports have in fact suggested that a substance found in grape skins has a beneficial effect on the lipoproteins profile. (Skins are included in the production of red but not white wine.) Actually red wine is only one of many differences between the French and American diets. Here are several others.

The French use more butter than Americans, (great quantities in northern France and less toward the south where olive oil is the main fat staple). They eat three times as much cheese and also use more cream. On the other hand, they drink only half the homogenized milk. They eat bread with every meal, but do not butter it. Butter is used primarily in cooking and baking and not as a solid spread, as it is in the United States and in Scandinavian countries.

Americans eat more than ten times as much refined sugar. Even though rich pastries are identified with France, the French tend to eat fruit and cheese at the end of a meal and save the rich desserts for special occasions.

Aside from specific foods, there are other differences as well. Food in France is more likely to be fresh than food bought in American supermarkets. Vegetables are often picked, sold, and eaten on the very same day. Bread may be purchased fresh before each meal. There is certainly less canned, frozen, vacuum-packed, shrink-wrapped, or cold-storaged food.

There are also lifestyle differences. The main meal in France is often taken at midday, in leisurely fashion, and followed by a rest period. Wine, whether red or white, is served *with* the meal, as opposed to the practice of drinking alcoholic beverages *before* meals. The French also take longer vacations. On the other hand, they smoke more and exercise less. Incidentally, even in France individuals with high risk factors are more likely to have heart attacks than those with better profiles.

In summary, a glass or two of wine, taken with a leisurely meal, seems to be beneficial. *More* than two drinks a day cancel out some of the benefits by increasing mortality from other causes. Other components of the French and American diets may sort themselves out in the coming years as Americans eat more prudently, while the French increasingly resort to fast foods, fast meals, more snacks, and less wine.

The Mediterranean region has a particularly good record with regard to heart disease. The ancient Greeks ate a healthful diet, and so do the present inhabitants of Greece, Italy, southern France, and Spain. Here too red wine is a common beverage. Crete has the lowest rate of heart attacks in Europe, and people there live the longest. The people of Crete consume large quantities of vegetables and grains including bread and pasta, and eat some fish and very little meat. Forty percent of their calories come from fat, which is more than what is currently recommended, but the fat is almost entirely olive oil. (It is said that some old-timers drink a small glass of olive oil for breakfast.) Families tend to eat together three times a day.

The Japanese have few heart attacks and the highest life expectancy in the world despite the notable incidence of high blood pressure and strokes, perhaps related to high salt intake. This picture may be changing. Fat consumption has tripled in the last few decades, as the classic meals of rice and vegetables have become less popular. What has gained most in popularity is fast food, especially in the cities and among the young. (More than a thousand McDonald's have sprung up in Japan.) One favorable change has been a drop in salt use. Smoking, however, goes on unabated. Along with their affluence and dietary westernization, the Japanese have gotten taller and fatter. Another decade or two will reveal if there are any more *serious* consequences. Japanese living in the United States have already narrowed the gap with regard to heart attacks and longevity.

The American diet has also undergone many changes. Fifty-odd years ago meat, eggs, milk, and dairy products were major components of the recommended diet. Over the ensuing decades fats, meats, eggs, and sugar were gradually de-emphasized and the stress is now on complex carbohydrates—bread, pasta, grains, fruits and vegetables. The Food Guide Pyramid shown below shows the current recommendations.

It is interesting that a century ago W. A. Atwater of the Agriculture

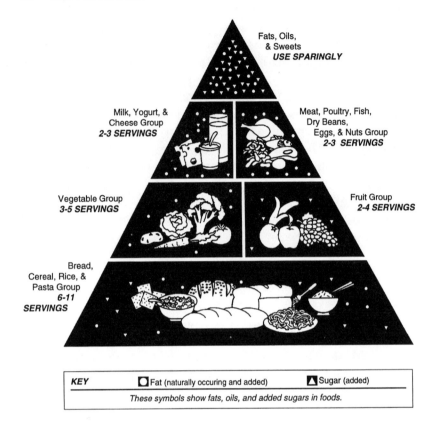

Department proposed a diet consisting of 52 percent of calories from carbohydrates, 33 percent from fat and 15 percent from protein. This is very close to current guidelines.

Despite all the health education, discussion of risk, and societal pressures, Americans have grown fatter over the years. This is due largely to poor eating habits, but also in part to a sedentary life style and lack of regular exercise.

Thirty percent of the population can be classified as obese (20 percent above upper limit of desirable weight). The average adult American has gained eight pounds in the last decade; the number of obese people has increased 25 percent. An estimated 300,000 deaths a year are attributed to obesity.

Obesity is a risk factor for cardiovascular disease, as well as for diabetes and hypertension, which themselves contribute to cardiovascular disease. Other relationships between diet and risk of disease (as acknowledged by the FDA) are (1) a salt and high blood pressure connection; (2) an increased risk of coronary heart disease related to a high saturated fat and cholesterol intake versus a decreased risk with a high fiber diet (especially soluble fiber); and (3) an increased likelihood of cancer associated with a high fat diet as contrasted to a decreased risk with a diet rich in grains, fruits, and vegetables. Other relationships have been suggested and are being studied.

It is beyond the scope of this book to recommend specific diets except to suggest that they include a variety of foods, with an emphasis on vegetables, fruits, and grain products; moderation in the use of salt and alcohol; and minimal use of fat and sugar. Gimmicky diets are usually unsuccessful over the long term.

CHAPTER 7
Familiar Subjects

We take it for granted that we know a lot about these topics because we deal with most of them every day. Nevertheless, closer examination may reveal some of the finer points.

WATER

It provides no calories, and may not always be to everyone's taste, but water is one substance we cannot live without. There is no cell, tissue, or organ that does not require water for normal functioning. Life as we know it cannot exist in its absence.

Our bodies are one-half to two-thirds water. In a 150-pound individual, that's about ten gallons. Depending on body size, activity, dietary factors, and climate, the daily turnover is usually between two and four quarts. In hot weather, with exercise, as much as fifteen quarts may be lost in a day. Too much water (within reason) is readily excreted, but an inadequate intake is hazardous, and can be more rapidly fatal than the lack of any other nutrient.

Water is obtained from food as well as from liquids. Some foods, especially fruits and vegetables, have a very high water content. Peaches, pears, oranges, and apples are up to 85 or 90 percent water; green beans, peppers, lettuces, cabbages, squashes, and several other vegetables have an even higher water content. In an average diet at least a third of the water we consume comes from "solid" food.

The excretion of water is handled mainly by the kidneys in the form of urine, but water is also lost as sweat through the skin, in the air exhaled through the lungs, and in the stool.

Water varies widely in mineral content. "Soft" water is relatively mineral-free; it makes nice suds and leaves little deposit. "Hard" or mineral-rich water is often tastier, and may or may not be better for your health depending on the minerals in it. As a rule, if a water softener is to be installed, it is best to attach it only to the hot water pipes, 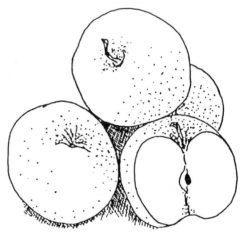 which supply water for bathing and laundry, and leave the minerals in the cold water for drinking, cooking, and outdoor chores.

Water must be monitored regularly, regardless of its source, because it may contain disease-causing bacteria and chemical pollutants (arsenic, benzene, nitrates, nitrites, lead, and radioactive substances). Boiling kills bacteria and parasites, but does not remove chemicals. Even distilled water may not be entirely pure; it also tends to be tasteless.

Bottled water, usually obtained from springs, contains varying amounts of minerals. When the concentration of minerals is above a certain level, the water is considered a "mineral water," whether the mineral content is natural or adjusted by the bottler. Similarly, in sparkling water, the carbonation (carbon dioxide gas) may come from a spring or may be introduced by the company.

Bottled water has become big business, partly for reasons of taste but partly also because some consumers don't trust their water supply. Bottled spring water, however, can be contaminated and polluted just like other water sources, and must be monitored regularly.

A large industry has sprung up around home water purification. Several systems are in common use. Reverse osmosis machines and high-volume carbon filters remove many contaminants, but bacteria and some toxic chemicals may remain. Faucet filters are usually inadequate, unless contamination is minimal. When safety, rather than taste, is a concern, it is best to rely on the findings of an independent lab (mail-order if necessary), or on data from the local utility company rather than on information provided by a company that sells purification equipment.

MILK

A great variety of milks is available to consumers. The following outline gives some of the types and their characteristics.

Whole milk: cow's milk that contains a minimum of 3¼ percent milk fat (butter fat) and a minimum of 8¼ percent nonfat milk solids.

Homogenized milk: milk that has been pumped under pressure through tiny holes of a homogenizer. The process reduces the size of fat globules and maintains an even distribution of fat throughout the liquid.

Pasteurized milk: milk that has been heated to 145 degrees for 30 minutes or to 158 degrees for 15 seconds; this destroys most organisms, particularly disease-causing bacteria and fungi.

Ultrapasteurized milk: milk that has been heated to about 285 degrees (well above the boiling point, but without boiling), for about three seconds. This process of Ultra High Temperature conservation (UHT) not only pasteurizes, but also increases the milk's shelf life up to six months, and obviates the need for refrigeration during storage.

Acidophilus milk: whole milk to which bacteria have been added that help digest lactose.

Raw milk: unpasteurized, unprocessed milk. Because of the danger of bacterial contamination, raw milk is considered unsafe and is banned by many states. Some states do permit raw milk if it is produced and certified by supervised dairies.

Low-fat milk: pasteurized milk whose fat content has been reduced to 1 percent. By FDA standards 2 percent milk does not qualify as a low-fat product, because it has more than 3 gm of fat per 8 oz serving; it does, however, have 40 percent less fat than whole milk, and 19 percent fewer calories.

Skim or non-fat milk: milk whose fat content has been reduced to less than ½ percent.

Evaporated milk: ultrapasteurized homogenized whole milk from which about 60 percent of the water has been removed.

Evaporated skim milk: skim milk with about 60 percent of the water removed.

Condensed sweetened milk: evaporated milk combined with a quantity of sugar, usually sucrose.

Dry (powdered) whole milk: pasteurized whole milk from which all water has been removed.

Non-fat dry (powdered) milk: pasteurized skim milk from which all water has been removed.

Cultured buttermilk: pasteurized low-fat milk in which bacteria have been cultured to create the characteristic taste of buttermilk.

Imitation milk: milk from which all milk fat has been removed and replaced by other fats or oils so that cholesterol content is minimized. The product may contain highly saturated oils.

Human milk (breast milk): Ounce for ounce, human milk contains slightly less protein and more cholesterol, fat, and calories than cow's milk. It has considerably less vitamin D than fortified cow's milk or commercial soy formulas. Quite uniquely, about 10 percent of the unsaturated fatty acids in breast milk is of the omega-3 variety.

Human milk contains several other substances lacking or deficient in cow's milk. Some, such as choline, inositol, and taurine are now being added to infant formulas. Others, for example carnitine, are being studied and considered for addition.

Breast milk possibly imparts to the infant a degree of protection against some infectious diseases and allergies. It can also transfer substances that are not desirable and may be hazardous. Narcotics, tranquilizers, alcohol, nicotine, and many medications, including some antibiotics and laxatives, are excreted in breast milk and may affect the nursing infant.

Soybean-based infant formula and soybean milk: soybean products used when milk is to be avoided for reasons of digestive problems, allergy, or vegetarianism.

Goat milk: usually not pasteurized, not licensed, and, like other raw milk, not safe. Pasteurized or not, goat milk has a higher fat content and more calories than cow's milk.

Lactose: the sugar naturally present in the milk of mammals.

Casein: milk protein, a standard for measuring the nutrient characteristics of other proteins.

CALORIE AND FAT CALORIE CONTENT OF DIFFERENT MILK VARIETIES

	Calories (per 8 oz)	Calories from Fat (per 8 oz)
Whole milk	150	72
homogenized		
pasteurized		
ultrapasteurized		
raw		
reconstituted dry whole milk		
imitation milk		
Two percent milk	121	42
One percent milk	102	23
Cultured buttermilk	100	20
Skim or non-fat milk	86	2
Half & Half	324	255
Light cream	504	445
Heavy cream	835	806
Evaporated whole milk	338	171
Evaporated skim milk	200	7
Condensed sweetened milk	980	238
Human milk	180	94
Goat milk	168	91
Soybean-based infant formula (avg.)	165	80
Liquid non-dairy creamer (avg.)	320	215

ALCOHOL

References to alcohol are found in some of our earliest records. The cultivation of grapes is depicted on Egyptian tomb paintings, and remnants of vines from 4000 B.C. have been discovered in Central Europe. Then as now, alcohol was used for medicinal and ritual purposes as well as for its pleasurable effects. Most fruits and grains and many vegetables were found to be fermentable, and spirits of all sorts were produced. Nevertheless, excessive use of alcohol is frowned upon by almost all societies. Some religions forbid it entirely.

Investigators say that one or two drinks a day help prevent heart attacks. A greater amount of alcohol fails in this regard. In addition, it displaces food and nutrients in the diet, reduces appetite, contributes to hypertension, and disturbs digestion and metabolism; ultimately, through toxic effects on the liver, chronic heavy use causes malnutrition and can lead to serious, even fatal, liver damage.

Although alcohol in all its forms is a central nervous system depressant, it is initially perceived to be a stimulant because it first tends to depress an individual's inhibitory centers, thus lessening tension and allowing for more relaxed behavior and communication. At the same time, mood control and judgment are impaired, and there is an escalating loss of mental and physical abilities as the blood alcohol level rises. Generally speaking, the "stronger" the drink, the more calories per ounce of liquor. Pure 100 percent alcohol provides seven calories per gram, less than fat but more than protein or carbohydrate. Eighty proof liquor (which is 40 percent alcohol) has less than three calories per gram. Mixers, while diluting the strength per ounce, may add calories to the whole. One drink of a jigger (1½ oz) of straight liquor, a can of beer, or five ounces of wine have about the same intoxicating effect, but beer has the most calories. Light beer has fewer calories than regular beer but the alcohol content is about the same. The following list compares (approximately) various representative alcoholic drinks with regard to calories and alcohol content.

	Amount (oz)	Calories	Alcohol (gm)
GIN, VODKA, WHISKEY, RUM			
80-proof	1½	104	15
LIQUEURS (cordials)	1	100	7
BRANDY, COGNAC	1	70	10
COCKTAILS			
Manhattan	3½	165	20
Martini	3½	140	19
Daiquiri	3½	131	15
Old-fashioned	4	180	24
WINES			
Table, red or white	5	105	13
Champagne	5	106	14
Aperitif (dry sherry)	2	85	9
Dessert (port)	3½	135	16
BEER			
Standard	12	150	15
Light beer	12	100	13
Nonalcoholic beer	12	68	1

Alcohol blood levels serve to confirm alcohol consumption and to determine the degree of intoxication. The following guidelines may be used:

Percentage of Blood Alcohol	State of Intoxication
.01 to .04	Evidence of drinking
.05 to .09	May be drunk
.10 to .14	Drunk
.15 and higher	Dead-drunk

For the purpose of defining "driving while intoxicated" (DWI), most states use 0.09 percent as the legal upper limit of acceptable blood alcohol. On the average, the body is able to metabolize about ten grams of pure alcohol, or slightly less than an ounce of 80 proof liquor, in an hour. The speed of drinking, therefore, plays a role in the degree of intoxication. Non-alcoholic men are able to dispose of alcohol more readily than women or than chronic alcoholics of either sex.

For a gross estimate of blood alcohol levels, the following chart may be used. It is based on body weight and on the amount of alcohol consumed on an empty stomach in a one-hour period.

BLOOD ALCOHOL LEVELS
(PERCENT ALCOHOL IN BLOOD)

80 proof (oz)	Wine (oz)	Beer (cans)	Body Weight (pounds)					
			120	140	160	180	200	220
2	7	1½	.07	.06	.05	.04	.04	.03
3	10	2	.10	.09	.08	.07	.06	.05
4	13	3	.13	.12	.10	.09	.08	.07
5	17	3	.17	.14	.13	.11	.10	.09
6	20	4	>.20	.17	.15	.13	.12	.11
7	23	5		>.20	.18	.16	.14	.13
8	27	5			>.20	.19	.16	.15
9	30	6				>.20	.18	.17
10	33	7					>.20	.19
11	37	7						>.20

Note: > = more than

CAFFEINE

Coffee plants have been grown for their stimulative properties for over a thousand years. Coffee is a newcomer, however, when compared to tea which has been cultivated for at least 3,000, and possibly 5,000 years. Both arrived in Europe in the seventeenth century, coffee from the Middle East and tea from the Far East.

Caffeine, an active ingredient in both beverages, has medicinal effects. Its stimulant properties are real. It promotes alertness and counteracts fatigue; thinking becomes clearer and manual skills are improved. In most adults the stimulant effects are mild and pleasurable. In children and in sensitive individuals, or when taken in excess, there may be adverse effects on the heart and nervous system manifested by rapid or irregular heart-beat, trembling, anxiety, and insomnia. Some of these effects can carry over to the unborn fetus or the breast-feeding infant. Pregnant and lactating women should therefore limit their caffeine intake.

Detractors claim that coffee increases cancer risk, causes fibrocystic breast disease, infertility and birth defects, raises cholesterol, and leads to high blood pressure. None of this has ever been found true in humans, although adverse effects have been observed in laboratory animals on very high doses of caffeine. There *is* evidence, however, that women who drink two or more cups of coffee daily during their adult lives increase their risk of osteoporosis in later life unless they have also consumed milk or taken a calcium supplement all along.

Coffee may aggravate ulcer symptoms. This is equally true for decaffeinated coffee; obviously, gastric irritants other than caffeine are involved. All types of coffee and tea should be avoided if they cause gastrointestinal problems.

Caffeine is addictive. In habitual users caffeine is needed for normal functioning. When it is stopped abruptly, withdrawal symptoms may occur for several days manifested by mental and physical sluggishness, headaches, and irritability.

Listed below are ranges of caffeine content in some common products. The exact amount varies with different

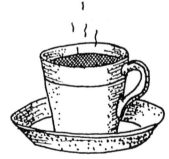

brands, methods of manufacture, and preparation. For those who avoid caffeinated beverages for themselves or their children, it should be pointed out that some *non*cola drinks may contain consideable amounts of caffeine.

Beverages	Caffeine (mg)
Coffee, 5 oz	60–100
Tea, 5 oz	20–110
Decaffeinated coffee or tea, 5 oz	1–5
Hot cocoa, 5 oz	4–25
Chocolate milk, 8 oz	2–7
Cola drinks, 12 oz	30–50
Diet colas, 12 oz	30–50
Decaffeinated cola drinks, 12 oz	1–10
Mountain Dew, 12 oz	about 70
Sunkist orange soda, 12 oz	about 35

Foods	
Coffee ice cream 2/3 cup	60–95
Coffee yogurt 1 cup	30–50
Baking chocolate, 1 oz	25–35
Dark chocolate, 1 oz	5–35
Milk chocolate, 1 oz	1–15
Chocolate syrup, 1 oz	5

Drugs (per standard dose)	
Anacin	64
Excedrin Extra Strength	130
No Doz	200
Vanquish	66
Vivarin	200

CHAPTER 8

Safety Issues and Controversies

Unlike the previous chapters, which deal with established information, some topics in this group are likely to provoke strong differences of opinion. Still, it is worthwhile to separate facts from myths to the best of our ability.

ORGANIC FOOD

The health food industry and its customers use the term "organic" to denote produce that was grown without chemical fertilizers or pesticides. Unless it is certified by a supervising agency, however, there is no guarantee that the claim is valid. Individual states define "organic" differently. Some require a minimum of three years between the last chemical application and the time of harvest. Others allow the term "organic," but set no guidelines on time. More than half the states are not concerned with definitions at all and set no rules.

Organic produce may be two or three times as expensive as its supermarket counterpart. The same is true for meat from animals that were raised "organically," that is, with no chemicals by injection or in the feed.

Chemical fertilizers, when properly constituted and applied, are generally not a health hazard. As a matter of fact, artificial fertilizer can sometimes be tailor-made to supply a mineral or other substance in which that particular soil is deficient. All things being equal, organi-

99

cally and nonorganically grown plants have the same nutritional value, taste, and appearance. Unfortunately conditions are *not* always equal and the use of chemicals, though legislated, cannot be monitored all of the time. Plants *can* pick up and retain unwanted substances when they are applied in excess and, aside from damaging the produce, these chemicals can also kill wildlife and pollute the water tables.

Most organic growers *do* avoid the use of chemicals—fertilizers, pesticides, herbicides, fungicides, fumigants—but what assurances do we have? (Incidentally, one would almost have to farm on virgin territory in a remote part of the world not to be affected by chemical contaminants, whether these substances are brought in by wind or water, or left behind from previous treatments. But, in the present context, such contamination is a nonissue.)

At this point the consumer must evaluate whatever information is available, and make the decision. Theoretically at least, there is no denying the appeal of organic farming. Whether it can fully succeed in an environment of industrial pollution and acid rain is another question. And it is equally questionable whether organic farming can produce maximum amounts of food in a world that has to deal with famines, depleted soil, and vanishing farmland. The hope must lie in new technologies.

"HEALTH FOODS," HEALTH FOOD SUPPLEMENTS, AND "NATURAL FOODS"

Over the past several decades we have made great strides in the science of nutrition, and the public has become much more aware of the importance of a healthful diet. For a variety of reasons there is also a growing tendency toward self-diagnosis and self-treatment.

Unfortunately, along with this burgeoning interest, increasing numbers of self-styled nutrition authorities and health food advocates have come on the scene, many with fancy (though meaningless) titles and degrees and most of them more skilled in salesmanship and oratory than in science. In recent years another source of misinformation has been added: irresponsible, misguided, and self-serving "experts" who hold forth on the Internet and on-line services, some of them ignorant and others, sales people in disguise, with a clear conflict of interest.

All of us want to eat foods that promote good health, but some foods and supplements make more sense than others. Fortunately current labeling laws will not permit unsubstantiated health claims.

Alfalfa, important as animal fodder, is promoted for its mineral, vitamin, and chlorophyll content. It is however largely indigestible by humans.

Bee pollen is the tiny male seed found in blossoms. The commercial product may also contain nectar (plant secretions) and bee saliva. Bee pollen has been advocated as a treatment for sterility, hardening of the arteries, poor muscle tone, etc. These claims have never been substantiated by any scientific studies. Undeniably bee pollen contains amino acids, vitamins, and minerals, but it is a very expensive source of nutrients that are readily available elsewhere.

Bioflavonoids: see flavonoids.

Bone meal is a mineral supplement that features large doses of calcium and other components of crushed or ground-up bone. It is not recommended because the product often contains unwanted contaminants, including lead.

Brewer's yeast (debittered, non-leavening yeast) can serve as a source of B vitamins, amino acids, and minerals, but it offers no advantage over other foods that contain these nutrients. One tablespoon has about twenty-five calories.

Carob is obtained from the pod of a Mediterranean tree. It is used as a substitute for chocolate because it has less fat and is free of stimulants. Incorporated in a candy bar, however, it is combined with other ingredients and ends up with a fat and calorie content similar to that of chocolate.

Chlorophyll plays an important role in plant metabolism but serves no nutritional function in humans. It is promoted as an internal deodorant.

DNA and RNA, ribonucleic acids, are specific and integral components of all cells, both animal and vegetable. Supplements, however, are not utilized and are useless.

Dolomite is a mineral supplement derived from limestone. It is rich in calcium and magnesium but measurements are not accurate or dependable. Dolomite may also include hazardous impurities, such as lead.

Flavonoids (or *bioflavonoids*) are substances found in plant foods, mostly in the rinds. They are reputed to supplement the actions of vitamin C. *Hesperidin,* from citrus fruit, and *rutin,* usually from buckwheat, are the best known among them. Along with *Acerola C,* a berry, and *rose hips,* the nodules under rose buds, they are variously grouped together as vitamin C complex or vitamin P. Bioflavonoids can also be derived from algae. The claims notwithstanding, flavonoids have not been shown to play a role in human nutrition.

Garlic is a very ancient folk remedy, believed to ward off disease as well as vampires, and to treat a variety of bites and other afflictons. Garlic may in fact have beneficial health effects. There is no hard evidence so far, but reputable researchers are investigating garlic and its many components for medicinal properties. 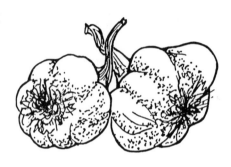 Studies so far suggest that garlic may lower cholesterol, reduce blood pressure, and diminish clot formation. Whatever its merits, there is no certainty yet that garlic is active when the odorous part is removed

Ginseng is a Chinese herb whose root is reputed to have the power to restore natural balance and sexual potency. Ginseng can cause diarrhea, nervousness, insomnia, and an increase in blood pressure. Its hormonal effects can be damaging to the unborn fetus and the use of ginseng is inadvisable during pregnancy.

Granola is a tasty non-specific combination of ingredients, among them oats, wheat germ, honey, brown sugar, coconut, raisins, nuts, seeds, and spices. It is usually high in calories and fat. Depending on the exact composition, two-thirds cup of granola can provide more than 350 calories, half of which may come from fat. Low-fat granola cereal has 210 calories per two-thirds cup.

Honey is probably the oldest cultivated sweetener, used throughout the ages. Except for some minerals, present in very small amounts, honey offers no nutritional advantage over table sugar, especially in the quantities that are ordinarily used. Raw honey should never be given to small children because it can cause very severe illness (a form of botulism). Adults are not susceptible to this toxin, but can have adverse reactions, if the bees have fed on poisonous plants.

Kelp is a supplement produced from seaweed. It is a rich source of iodine and also of magnesium and calcium. It may also contain harmful amounts of arsenic.

Macrobiotics are various cereal grains. A true macrobiotic diet is nutritionally incomplete. Macrobiosis actually means "longevity," but long life is not furthered by a deficient diet.

Megavitamins are very large doses of vitamins with amounts far greater than required for good nutrition or for the prevention of deficiency. Some megavitamins are useless, but harmless; some are toxic, particularly megadoses of vitamins A and D, and some, while not toxic in themselves, may interfere with the utilization of other nutrients.

Since vitamins are used by the body in trace amounts, megadoses don't make sense. Or do they? The topic is of great interest, and is discussed further in the section "Free Radicals and Antioxidants."

Natural is not a meaningful term when applied to food because there are no standards of definition. And being natural doesn't necessarily make a substance desirable in one's food.

Papain (papase) is an enzyme found in papaya. Because it breaks down protein, it is used to tenderize tough cuts of meat, but it is useless when taken as a tablet.

Royal jelly is a substance secreted by worker bees to promote the development of the queen bee. It does nothing for human beings.

Vegetarianism that permits eggs and dairy products (lacto-ovo vegetarianism) allows for an adequate protein intake, but may be high in saturated fat and cholesterol. Prepared vegetarian foods, such as fettucine Alfredo, macaroni and cheese, and even vegetable lasagna contain considerable amounts of fat.

Strict vegetarians who avoid all animal products must be circumspect about getting enough protein and vitamin B_{12}.

Vitamin B_{12} injections are worthless in healthy individuals who eat a varied diet.

Wheat germ, a portion of the wheat seed, is a rich source of vitamin E. It also supplies some minerals and B vitamins. An ounce of toasted wheat germ has 108 calories, 25 percent of them from fat.

HERBS AND HERBAL TEAS, ROOTS AND BARKS

Starting with the most ancient civilizations, herbs have been used for their medicinal properties. Our oldest written document, the Ebers papyrus, dated at 3500 years old, contains a description of herbal treatments. Many subsequent cultures produced elaborate and comprehensive treatises on medicinal plants, known as herbals; and some present-day societies still depend on the healing powers of herbs.

Many plants do indeed have potent medicinal properties—among them foxglove, belladonna, and henbane. In many instances the active ingredients have been identified and can now be synthesized. Manufactured drugs are safer than extracts of plants: they can be produced without impurities, they are uniform and of predictable strength, and they are subjected to extensive testing and quality controls. The majority of herbs has not undergone acceptable safety and efficacy testing. There are numerous reports of toxic effects, particularly involving the liver; some cases have been fatal and a few have required liver transplants. It is possible that some instances of "hepatitis" are actually due to adverse effects of herbs. Among those that have been identified as potential liver toxins are chaparral, comfrey, germander, Jin Bu Huan and skullcap. Self-treatment with any such plant products is very unwise.

Herbal teas pose a related problem. They are promoted for being *natural* products (so are poisonous mushrooms, tobacco and various drugs of abuse), and for being free of stimulants. Some herbal teas, in fact, do contain significant amounts of caffeine. More important, they can be health hazards in several ways: medicinal ingredients in the tea may produce unexpected and undesirable side effects; the herbs could have been sprayed or contaminated with toxic chemicals (supervision is often poor); and allergic reactions are not uncommon (chamomile, for instance, is related to ragweed). Herbal teas should be used only if marketed by a reputable company.

There are literally thousands of plants that have been used for medicinal or mystical reasons. Some with truly dangerous potential are classified as poisonous plants. Mentioned here, alphabetically, are some of the better known herbs, roots, barks, etc., all available in stores or by mail order. They can be harmful, particularly when used by pregnant women, when given to the very young or old, when taken in excess, or when substituted for conventional medicine to treat an illness. Here is a selection:

HERBS, ROOTS, AND BARKS
Promoted as Health Foods

achuma	dong quai	ma hueng
aconite	echinacea	mandrake
agrimony	elecampane	mohudu
akee	euphorbia	monkshood
aloe vera	eyebright	mullein
angelica	fenugreek	pau d'arco
astragulus	feverfew	pennyroyal
baneberry	fritilleria	polygala tenuifolia
biloba	gentian	probolis
black cohosh	germander	quassia
blackberry leaf	ginkgo leaf	rue
bloodroot	ginseng (see	saffron
blue flag	Health Foods)	sarsaperilla
boneset	golden seal	sassafras
borage	gotu-kola	schizandra
burdock root	guarana	seawrack
cananga	hellebore	skullcap
castor	ho shou wu	slippery elm
catnip	horsetail	snake root
chamomile	hyssop	soksi
chaparral	iboga	spirulina (an alga)
chickweed	Iceland moss	squaw vine
cleavers	ipe roxo	St. John's wort
colts foot	Jin Bu Huan	taheebo
comfrey	jojoba	thistle
culebra	kava kava	valerian
damiana	lantana	vervein
dandelion	licorice	yarrow
	lobelia	

FREE RADICALS AND ANTIOXIDANTS

Free radicals are the extra unpaired electrons found on some molecules. Such a molecule becomes very active trying to find another molecule to which the electron can attach itself. Not only will this damage the new found molecule, but it can start a chain reaction as the new unbalanced molecule seeks yet another recipient.

Oxygen radicals are the most common culprits. They can be created by ozone, X-rays, industrial emissions, and other environmental onslaughts. They can be found in food and within our bodies as the result of normal reactions. The healthy organism can usually rid itself of these radicals, but even the healthiest may not be able to deal with a massive assault such as that produced by heavy X-radiation. Air pollution, smoking, pesticides, viruses, chemicals, improper food storage and handling (heating fats too hot or too often), and unfiltered sunlight have all been implicated in the formation of free radicals. Free radicals are suspected of playing a role in the causation of many disorders: cancer, hardening of the arteries, autoimmune diseases such as rheumatoid arthritis and lupus, cataracts, and possibly Alzheimer's disease as well as the whole aging process.

Antioxidants by definition delay or prevent oxidation and it stands to reason that they can counteract free radicals, which are "oxidants." By blocking these free radicals and rendering them harmless as it were, antioxidants are intended to protect tissues from damage.

Advocates of antioxidants claim that they prevent damage from pollution, help cardiac patients to ward off further impairment, and retard the formation of cataracts and other tissue damage associated with aging.

Vitamins A, C, and E and selenium are the nutrients believed to have significant antioxidant activity. When given at antioxidant doses, these compounds should be considered drugs rather than supplements. Advocates recommend 1000 to 3000 mg of vitamin C, 100 to 800 mg of vitamin E, 10,000 to 90,000 USP of beta-carotene, and 100 to 200 mcg of selenium. Several other nutrients and drugs are also being studied for their antioxidant properties.

Specific groups of people may be more in need of antioxidant vitamins than others. Smokers require extra vitamin C and consumers of large amounts of unsaturated fatty acids need more vitamin E. But even without these specific risk factors more and more people, many scientists among them, take antioxidants daily. There are several responsible studies that support this concept. Nevertheless after decades of random megadosing, the evidence is not conclusive and there is no scientific proof that antioxidants contribute to a healthier or longer life. It will take more controlled clinical trials over longer periods of time before definite conclusions can be drawn.

IRRADIATION OF FOOD

Food irradiation is a very effective method of combating some serious agricultural problems: the bacterial contamination of meat, poultry, and seafood, the insect infestation of grains, nuts, and spices and the sprouting and too rapid ripening of vegetables and fruits. Irradiation is not used much, however, because the public is wary if not downright opposed to the concept. The process is also very expensive. More than a dozen countries have approved the irradiation of poultry to prevent bacterial disease. In the United States, where it has been permitted since 1992, the process has not been utilized to any extent by the large poultry companies.

On the part of the public the main objections to irradiation are safety issues: the possible changes within the molecules of the food stuff, particularly the creation of free radicals, and the destruction of vitamins. There is also the fear that resistant bacteria might survive and flourish. In any event, viruses will not be eliminated, and neither will toxins that were produced by bacteria prior to irradiation (the toxin that produces botulism, for example). Some opponents also suggest that irradiation might be used as a substitute for cleanliness and meticulous processing.

It is interesting that several of these objections were also raised when the pasteurization of milk was first advocated decades ago. It must also be said that no apparent harm came to astronauts or to American troops in Vietnam who ate irradiated meals, and no untoward effects have been demonstrated in animals given irradiated feed. What's more, some alternative substances or methods used to increase shelf life such as various chemicals, insecticides, preservatives, or intense heat carry their own adverse potentials.

Fresh food preserved by irradiation can survive long shipments and storage under less than perfect conditions. This could be a boon at times of natural catastrophe and in areas of malnutrition or famine.

Since 1958 the FDA has classified irradiation as a food additive. Under that heading its use must be approved for a specific food product and the product must be marked with the radiation logo, called a *radura,* which is a circle containing a flower with a dot above it. If, however, only an *ingredient* has been irradiated (such as mushrooms used for canned mushroom soup or strawberries used in jam), this fact need not be disclosed.

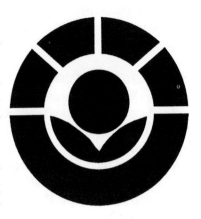

Consumers and legislators have work to do before irradiation assumes its rightful place in the food industry.

ADDITIVES

Natural and synthetic substances are added to foods for a variety of reasons. Some prevent spoilage and thereby add to the longevity of a product. Some maintain consistency and texture. Some add flavor, some add color, and some even improve the nutritional value by preventing vitamin loss.

Some additives must be listed on the label (nitrites, sulfites, tartrazine, etc.), some can be lumped together ("artificial colors and flavors"), and some don't have to be mentioned at all. In general, additives must be listed if they could be unsafe under certain conditions.

Many additives are used to prolong the shelf life of food products, but they also work in the consumer's interest. They inhibit mold formation on bread, and ice crystal formation in ice cream; they keep salt from caking and cake from tasting stale.

The list of additives in our food is almost endless; the number is actually in the thousands. We rely heavily on governmental agencies to oversee their use, and on consumer groups to press for continued testing. The FDA is entrusted with monitoring all additives with a computerized program called ARMS (Adverse Reaction Monitoring System).

There is no evidence that food additives cause hyperactivity in children.

Coloring agents could be considered frivolous additives because they are used primarily to make food look more appealing. Without them, many consumers would miss the dark caramel of cola drinks, the pretty pink of strawberry ice cream. and the pale yellow of butter and margarine. Butter was first colored 700 years ago. Consumers also associate the expected color with good quality. For example, oranges that are green could look unripe or inferior, even though that is not necessarily the case; for this reason, oranges are often colored orange.

"Certified colors" are manufactured and each batch is tested. Coloring agents that are derived from natural products, such as carrot oil or grape juice, need not be certified. Certified (synthetic) colors are often preferred because they do not impart a flavor of their own; they are also more stable and more versatile in achieving color gradations.

Preservatives keep foods from spoiling and also from tasting stale or rancid. Salt is the oldest and still the most commonly used preservative, particularly for meat and fish. Wherever refrigeration is not available, heavy salting is a tried and true alternative.

Well known among preservatives are *nitrites:* they not only preserve processed meats, but also intensify their color (bacon, hot dogs etc.). Although the body actually produces its own nitrites from nitrates in the diet (nitrates are abundant in vegetables), their safety has been questioned repeatedly, because under certain conditions nitrites react to form nitrosamines which are implicated in the development of some cancers. All in all, nitrite-rich foods are best limited, or avoided when there is a choice, especially by children.

Sulfites are another group of compounds involved in controversy. Starting with the Romans, who used sulfites to cleanse their wine containers, these substances have served to inhibit bacterial growth and delay deterioration of foods. In our day, however, their main use is often for appearance. When sprayed on fruits and vegetables, sulfites make these foods look fresh and attractive, even after prolonged exposure to air. This specific use of sulfites has been banned in salad bars, because in sensitive individuals sulfites can produce serious symptoms, including wheezing, rash, abdominal cramps, vomiting, and fainting. Salad bars are not a good idea anyway: there is too much opportunity for contamination.

Wine, beer, dried fruits, instant potatoes, soups and many other processed foods and drugs must be labeled with regard to sulfite content, so that sensitive individuals can avoid them. Wine bottled before 1988 will not be marked. Neither, of course, is restaurant food.

Sulfites are actually antioxidants, substances that protect foods from the specific hazards of oxygen, such as occurs with exposure to air. Other preservatives in this group are BHA and BHT; they too have been questioned with regard to safety. Antioxidants as a group are discussed elsewhere.

Humectants hold moisture and protect foods from drying out.

Anti-caking agents absorb moisture and allow powdered food to flow freely.

Emulsifiers keep substances mixed and uniform, even substances that normally don't mix at all, such as oil and water. Glycerides and lecithin are common examples. Emulsifiers are used in such products as salad dressings, peanut butter, and ice cream.

Sequestrants and **chelators** prevent substances, especially tiny amounts of metals, from mixing or interacting with foods, thereby spoiling or discoloring them.

Thickeners enhance the texture of such foods as yogurt and ice cream. Various gums and starches are commonly used.

Stabilizers prevent physical changes in ingredients, most notably the deterioration of flavors.

Flavor enhancers "bring out the flavor" in food. The chief one is MSG (monosodium glutamate), a substance used widely in commercial food processing. Many people report unpleasant side effects from MSG (the "Chinese restaurant syndrome"), but others deny that such a syndrome even exists. MSG contains a lot of sodium (salt). MSG should best be avoided by young children and used sparingly by adults.

Fortifiers are substances not normally present in a food product that are added to improve the nutrient value. The fortification of milk with vitamin D has had a major impact on the health of children. Some additions, however, increase the cost of a product without adding significantly to good nutrition.

PESTICIDES

In any discussion of food safety, the subject of pesticides is bound to be raised as an important issue. Broadly speaking the term *pesticide* denotes any material that is used to control insects, molds, diseases, and weeds. Almost a billion pounds of chemicals are used annually in the United States for this purpose.

The application of pesticides is intended to enhance the quality and quantity of farm products. Unfortunately, some chemicals are pervasive; not only do they coat the fruit or vegetable, but under some conditions they may enter the product itself, and no amount of washing will remove them. Even the surfaces cannot always be cleaned effectively, if the produce has been waxed, or coated with a chemical for the sake of appearance or preservation.

Nor does pervasiveness apply just to the produce for whose benefit it was intended! Chemical residue can be detected in meat, poultry, and fish, if these animals consumed pesticide-tainted vegetation. Even chemicals used on nonedible crops such as cotton can eventually pollute the water table and enter the food chain. And some pesticides stay around for a long time: DDT residue is still found in some crops, decades after it was banned!

So much for the bad news.

Chemical pesticides fulfill a need, particularly when food has to be mass-produced at reasonable cost. Insect plagues can destroy entire crops, and even milder infestations make food unacceptable to the consumer. The FDA spends twenty million dollars a year on pesticide monitoring, and has consistently found that 98% of all farm products sold have zero or very low levels of residue.

Much progress has been made in these areas: the public has become more educated and vocal, and several strong government agencies are committed to the safe and effective use of chemicals in agriculture, chief among them the Environmental Protection Agency (EPA) the Food and Drug Administration (FDA) and the U.S. Department of Agriculture. Government agencies regularly check the "market basket" for chemical residue. Nevertheless there are still many rough edges in monitoring pesticide residue. Imported prod-

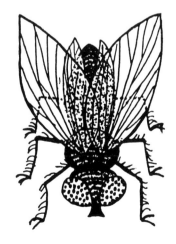

ucts are especially difficult to control, since only spot checks can be made. Foreign growers may not only apply more pesticides, but they could be using chemicals forbidden in the United States.

Fortunately, newer and safer means of pest control are being studied and developed. Certain planting techniques can shade out weeds effectively. Another trick lies in cultivating insect breeds that are harmless to food plants, but feed off the harmful insects. Bacteria and bacterial products have been in use for several years against some beetles, larvae and fungi. The use of pheromones is of great interest: the scents normally elaborated by female insects to attract males can be synthesized and placed in strategic areas to confuse the males and prevent reproduction

A natural virus has been employed in farming for half a century, but it is not specific enough, and can do damage to other plants. Specificity is very important The science of genetic engineering, may provide the answer. One genetically engineered virus has been approved, and it is hoped that this technology will create *specific* biological products that will be the natural enemies *of specific* pests, while being totally safe for man.

Genetic engineering may also succeed in creating crops that are more disease and pest resistant than their ancestors, and plants that can tolerate weed killers and other chemicals without damage to themselves or potential toxicity to the consumer. This is also one of the aims of scientific hybridization.

Without much doubt, chemicals will continue to be used, but here too there will be an increasing emphasis on specificity: using small amounts of the right stuff at the right time and place. As of now, fewer than 3 percent of all farmers in the United States farm entirely without the use of chemicals. Some farmers are actually discouraged from introducing better methods, such as crop rotation, because they are boxed into growing federally supported crops—wheat, corn, soybeans, and cotton—or lose their subsidies.

Consumer issues aside, chemical pesticides pose a particularly great hazard to farm workers. Migrant workers often live near pesticide-treated fields, along with their families, and safety rules are not always strictly enforced. They are exposed to pesticides in the air, and residue in the water and soil. Added to poor nutrition and poor sanitation, exposure to toxic chemicals makes migrant farm workers the highest risk group with regard to occupational illness.

HORMONES

Hormones are essential substances produced and secreted by specific glands of the body. Hormone-producing glands are known as ductless or endocrine glands, because they discharge their products directly into the blood stream, in contrast to exocrine glands which deliver their material to nearby areas, often by way of ducts: tears, saliva, sweat, etc.

The endocrine glands are the pituitary, thyroid, parathyroid, and adrenal glands, the sex glands (testes and ovaries) and the pancreas, which also plays an exocrine role.

Hormones serve vital functions with regard to metabolism, growth, sexual development, reproduction, and response to exercise and stress. For specific medical problems hormonal substances are prescribed; among these hormones are insulin, birth control pills, cortisone, and thyroid hormone.

Anabolic steroids ("steroids"), sometimes used and abused by athletes for muscle building, are a form of male sex hormone. An informal survey of football players showed that 10 to 25 percent of them had taken steroids. The percentage is undoubtedly even higher, particularly in some other sports, such as weight lifting. Steroids do build muscle tissue, but they also have serious side effects, possibly permanent, including liver damage, premature heart disease, sexual dysfunction, aggressive behavior and other psychological problems. In women they also produce acne, male type hair growth and hair loss, and deepening of the voice.

Growth hormone, a pituitary hormone, has *also* been used for muscle building, primarily because it is harder to detect than anabolic steroids. Unlike anabolic steroids, it may do more for the size of muscles than for their strength. Growth hormone is a valuable drug when used for the right reasons, but muscle building for athletic performance is not one of them.

As long as nutrition is not grossly impaired, such as in starvation or with extreme weight loss, and as long as there is an adequate source of iodine, hormone production is generally not affected by specific food intake. Contrary to what some people believe, obesity is very rarely due to a hormonal imbalance. It is in fact more likely to be the other way around: morbid obesity can cause hormone imbalance, and the same is true for excessive leanness.

The injection of a hormone or its addition to the feed of livestock and poultry is quite a different topic. The practice has been espoused by some, and severely criticized by others. Hormones and hormone-releasing substances can indeed enhance the quality and quantity of meat, making the animals grow faster and leaner.

Milk production can also be increased. Bovine somatotropin (BST) has been approved after extensive testing by governmental and private organizations. When injected into cows, BST boosts milk production as much as 20% without affecting the taste or composition of the milk.

Such practices have major economic consequences. Consumers, however, are less concerned with farm economics than with safety issues. Despite assurances by scientists and government agencies, uncertainties remain in the minds of the public about the use of hormones, particularly since the practice is not disclosed on the product in most states. (Vermont was the first state to enact a labeling law for BST treated milk, and several other states followed suit.) Consumers are wary and skeptical. Will there be more udder infections? Probably. Will antibiotics be given and will they show up in the milk? Probably not, since all milk is tested for antibiotic residue.

Also to be considered is the cost to dairy farmers, perhaps prohibitive for small family farms. Then there is the glut of milk to deal with, when there is already a surplus, and the tax burden of more dairy price support programs.

Ultimately the fate of BST will depend on acceptance by the public and other market forces.

CARNITINE (L-CARNITINE)

L-carnitine, once known as "vitamin B_T" and "B_T factor," is a substance normally present in liver and muscle tissue. It is not a vitamin, but plays a significant role in the transport of fatty acids. Beyond infancy, carnitine is supplied by the average diet, and is also synthesized from amino acids. Newborns, however, cannot synthesize sufficient amounts, and may become deficient if fed an unfortified soy formula.

Richest sources: Red meat
*   Milk, including powdered and skim*

Deficiency is very rare, but may occur as a genetic disease, and also with severe protein malnutrition, prolonged intravenous feeding or kidney dialysis. It is manifested by progressive muscle weakness.

L-carnitine is mentioned in this section because it has been promoted to athletes under the mistaken notion that it enhances energy and endurance by mobilizing fat from tissues. Some athletes are persuaded that it will substitute for anabolic steroids, and do less harm. While there has been some research that shows carnitine to increase the walking distance in individuals with very poor circulation, there is no such evidence in any controlled studies with athletes or other healthy people. Long-term effects of L-carnitine supplements are not known.

FOOD ALLERGIES

Food allergies affect one or two percent of adults. The allergies usually manifest themselves with skin problems. Sometimes the primary effect is on the respiratory or gastrointestinal tract. The foods most often responsible for allergic reactions in adults are fish, shellfish and nuts. In children the most common allergens are eggs, milk, peanuts, wheat and soy.

When allergy affects the skin, it can produce a rash, hives, puffiness and itching. Respiratory symptoms include sneezing, wheezing, congestion and runny nose. Full-blown asthmatic attacks may occur.

When the gastrointestinal tract is the primary target, allergy must be distinguished from food intolerance, such as an inability to digest milk, or some sort of intestinal disease. Symptoms with all these conditions may include cramps, nausea, vomiting, and diarrhea.

Elimination diets serve to make a diagnosis. Avoidance of the offending food is the best course of action, but this is not always easy, especially in the case of milk protein (casein) which is found in numerous processed foods.

FOOD POISONS

Proper food handling and food storage are the best prevention against food poisoning, even though we cannot always control all the variables.

It should be routine to wash fruits and vegetables thoroughly to remove insecticides, fungicides and any other chemicals that may have been applied to the surface. Even if the produce is to be peeled, it is advisable to wash it first. Detergent is not recommended. Unwashed fruit can be a particular, though rare, problem in commercial products. Unwashed peels, used in unpasteurized cider, for instance, pose a hazard.

Viruses, bacteria, and parasites actually produce far more illness than chemicals. The most common bacteria to cause food related illness are salmonella, campylobacter, E. coli and vibrio, and the most common cause of contamination is the exposure to fecal material during slaughter. Chicken and other poultry should always be washed, inside and out, and so should the surfaces that they have touched. Most important, poultry must be cooked to an internal temperature of 185°. Stuffing should be added just before cooking, because stuffing provides a good growth medium for bacteria from the poultry.

Bacterial and, in some instances, parasitic infestation can occur in all raw animal products. Much as we may enjoy steak tartare, sashimi, seviche, sushi, eggnog and Caesar salad, we must realize that eating raw meat, fish, and eggs carries a certain risk which is eliminated by cooking, or sometimes by prior freezing. The most hazardous foods of all are raw or undercooked mollusks.

Meat and poultry inspection by governmental agencies leaves a lot to be desired. Bacteria are not visible to the naked eye. It is well known that microscopic testing is much more valuable than inspection by looking, smelling and feeling. If consumer groups prevail and funding is made available, microscopic checks will be provided soon, along with stricter rules on cleanliness and temperature control.

Bacterial contamination is a serious problem. The total number of bacteria-caused illness is estimated at 6 1/2 million per year, with 9000 deaths. Half the illnesses and at least one fourth of the deaths are due to salmonella. E. coli bacteria in ground beef cause about 20,000 illnesses and 500 deaths annually. This problem can be prevented by thorough cooking.

Increasingly we also hear about toxic chemical contamination, particularly of fish, with substances such as dioxin and mercury. This is a problem that neither cooking nor freezing will solve. Only strong environmental legislation can help to prevent toxic pollution of oceans, lakes and streams.

Fish may also contain toxins unrelated to the pollution created by man. Chief among these is ciguatera toxin. Fish that feed on algae in tropical reefs, such as snapper, grouper, shark and amberjack, ingest this toxin which is not harmful to the fish, but causes illness in the consumer. Symptoms are gastrointestinal and then neurological, with marked disturbances of sensation. Another hazard is "red tide" (saxitoxin) which contaminates mollusks and causes paralytic shellfish poisoning, again with gastrointestinal and neurologic symptoms. Yet another gastrointestinal illness is scombroid fish poisoning, usually related to eating fish caught in open waters and then held at too high a temperature.

Some foods tell you that they are no longer safe, by their odor or change in appearance; consider them inedible. Bulging or leaking cans and cracked containers should be discarded without a taste test. Food that has been sitting out on a buffet table for hours is best avoided, as is perishable food on a summer camping trip when there is no refrigeration. In fact, in warm weather it is a good idea to bring a cooler to the supermarket, when the trip home is a long one.

Of all the safety measures over which we have control, perhaps the simplest one is hand washing, particularly before eating.

Food poisoning should always be reported to the local Health Department if the suspected source is a processed food product or a public eating place.

POISONOUS PLANTS

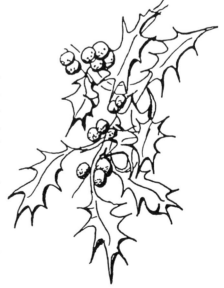

Poisoning from house and garden plants is not uncommon, especially among toddlers and young children. No one should taste any leaves, flowers, or berries, unless the plant is known to be safe. A poison control center should be called, when there is even a question about an unknown substance.

Eating poisonous plants can cause a variety of reactions, ranging from mild irritation in and around the mouth to severe illness that may involve almost every organ system.

Only non-foods are listed below (some under several different names). It should be remembered, however, that even common food plants can be toxic if the wrong part of the plant is consumed; potato sprouts are a prime example. Everyone knows, of course, that some mushrooms are extremely poisonous; their identification should never be left to amateurs.

Poisonous Shrubs, Flowers, Herbs, and Weeds

Absinth	Henbane	Periwinkle
Aesculus	High John root	Podophyllum
Apple of Peru	Hog's bean	Red puccoon
Arnica	Horse chestnut	Richweed
Asthma weed	Hyoscyamus	Saint Bennet's herb
Belladonna	Hypericum	St. John's wort
Bittersweet	Irish broom	Sanguinaria
Bleeding heart	Jack-in-the-pulpit	Scoparius
Bloodroot	Jalap	Scotch broom
Broom	Jimson weed	Snakeroot
Broomtop	Klamath weed	Spartium
Buckeye	Larkspur	Spindle tree
Burning bush	Leopard's bane	Spotted cowbane
Calamus	Lily of the valley	Stamonium
Conium	Lobelia	Sweet cane
Convallaria	Madderwort	Sweet cinnamon
Datura	Mandrake	Sweet flag
Devil's apple	May apple	Sweet root
Devil's eye	May lily	Thornapple
Dulcamara	Mingwort	Tobacco
Emetic Weed	Mistletoe	Tolguacha
Euonymus	Morning-glory	Tonka bean
Fool's Parsley	Mugwort	Umbrella plant
Foxglove	Myrtle	Wolf's bane
Goatweed	Nightshade*	Wormwood
Hemlock		Yohimbe

*Some nightshade plants should be excepted from this list: potatoes, tomatoes, peppers and eggplants among them. They are age-old important food crops, and not poisonous when eaten in normal amounts. However, the leaves of the tomato plant and the potato plant are very toxic, and so are potato shoots and green spots. Even potato skins in large amounts (1 or 2 lb) can cause serious illness.

Poisonous Houseplants

Caladium	Ivy	Oleander
Dieffenbachia	Jerusalem cherry	Philodendron
Elephant ear	Mistletoe	Poinsettia
Holly	Monstera	

Poisonous Bulbs

Amaryllis	Daffodil	Iris
Crocus	Hyacinth	Narcissus

CHAPTER 9
Miscellaneous Topics

As the heading says, this chapter deals with odds and ends, all connected with food in one way or another.

ENZYMES

Enzymes, defined as "organic catalysts," are substances that expedite chemical reactions in the body, without participating in the actual process. Innumerable different enzymes are needed for the innumerable processes that take place. With some exceptions, enzymes cannot be eaten. Specific body cells must produce specific enzymes for specific functions. The names of enzymes usually end with "ase."

Digestive enzymes, secreted in the mouth, stomach, pancreas and intestinal tract aid in the breakdown of the food we eat. Other enzymes help to convert sugars, fats, and amino acids into an appropriate form for energy use, tissue development, or storage. Enzymes play a role in nerve transmission, clotting, wound healing, and drug utilization—in fact, in almost every bodily activity.

LACTASE

Lactase is an enzyme normally found in the small intestine of mammals. It aids in the digestion of milk, specifically by breaking down lactose (milk sugar) into simpler sugars (glucose and galactose) that are suitable for absorption. Most humans, as well as other mammals, lose lactase activity as they grow into adulthood, and, with it, the ability to digest milk. The loss is much greater in some ethnic groups than in others. Evolutionary factors may play a role in these differences, since societies with a prominent dairy agriculture have a better genetic makeup for handling milk.

Ethnic Group	Approximate Percentage of Adults Affected by Lactase Deficiency
Northern Europeans	10
Mediterranean Europeans	75
Jews	80
African Americans	80
Native Americans	80
Asians	95
World population as a whole	70

Judged by mammalian standards, lactase deficiency is actually the more normal condition, because few adult animals drink milk. But, although growing up usually results in an intolerance to lactose, the deficiency is rarely complete, so that most people can tolerate small amounts of milk without discomfort. About 10 percent of the population, however, is sensitive to even the smallest quantities.

Skim milk, low fat milk, whole milk, and buttermilk (in that order) are most likely to cause difficulties. Yogurt, although high in lactose, contains an enzyme in its culture that aids in lactose digestion, so that symptoms are less common and less severe. (This is not true of frozen yogurt, because freezing destroys this enzyme.) The various other dairy products are rarely a problem. One would have to eat 10 ounces of processed cheese, or a stick of butter, or a cup of sour cream to consume the lactose found in 8 ounces of milk.

Symptoms of intolerance, when they occur, may variously consist of bloating, abdominal rumbling, cramps, nausea, flatulence, and diarrhea. The most effective way of avoiding discomfort is to limit lactose intake to one's tolerance level. When taken with a meal, milk is less likely to cause symptoms than when drunk by itself. For those who want to increase their milk intake beyond tolerance, commercial lactase may help a little. It can be taken along with the dairy product, or it may be added to the milk some hours ahead of time so that the lactose is predigested.

To avoid any possible confusion, it should be stated that lactase deficiency is quite different from a congenital and much more serious enzyme disorder, galactosemia, which precludes the normal metabolism of galactose, and which must be treated by avoidance of all dairy products and all foods and drugs containing even the smallest amounts of lactose.

TYRAMINE

Tyramine is a derivative of the amino acid tyrosine. Its significance lies chiefly in the effect it has on individuals who are taking monoamine oxidase (MAO) inhibitors, a group of drugs at times prescribed for depression or hypertension (high blood pressure). When a patient receives such a medication and then eats one of the tyramine-rich foods, severe and possibly life-threatening reactions may occur.

Listed below are foods and beverages that contain significant amounts of tyramine:

- Aged cheeses, such as brie, camembert, roquefort, stilton, blue, parmesan, Swiss and cheddar (Cream cheese and cottage cheese are safe.)
- Pickled, smoked and dried fish
- Smoked sausages, such as salami, bologna, pepperoni
- Liver
- Brewer's yeast
- Bananas, especially green bananas
- Fava beans (Italian broad beans)
- Avocado
- Yogurt
- Soy sauce
- Vanilla (except in minute amounts)
- Wine, especially Chianti and sherry, but others as well
- Beer and ale
- Chocolate

TAURINE

Taurine, a type of amino acid, participates in many metabolic processes. It plays a role in the formation of bile salts (the name "taurine" refers to ox bile) and also seems to be involved in activities of the heart and other organs under nervous control. Because the body can synthesize it from other amino acids, taurine is not considered essential in the diet.

Richest sources: Raw clams and oysters
Breast milk

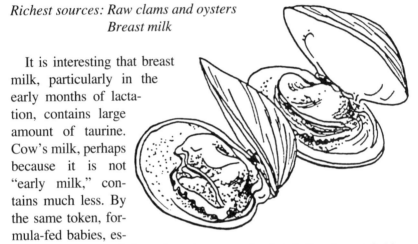

It is interesting that breast milk, particularly in the early months of lactation, contains large amount of taurine. Cow's milk, perhaps because it is not "early milk," contains much less. By the same token, formula-fed babies, especially premature infants, have lower taurine levels than breast-fed babies. Even at low levels, however, no deficiency effects have been demonstrated. Nevertheless, taurine is now being added to infant formulas, and consideration is being given to adding it to long-term intravenous feedings, particularly for infants.

ASH—ALKALINE AND ACID

The expressions acid ash and alkaline ash refer to the effect of a particular food on the acidity or alkalinity of urine after the food item has been metabolized. This is generally of importance only when it influences the effectiveness of a drug; some drugs require a certain urine pH (degree of acidity) to produce their desired effect on the urinary tract.

Interestingly, some foods we consider as acid tend to make the urine more alkaline; citrus fruits are an example.

Acid-ash foods include: meat, poultry, fish, shellfish, eggs, cheese, bread, pasta, cereal, cranberries and plums.

Alkaline-ash foods include: milk and dairy products (except cheese), almost all fruits, most vegetables, corn, legumes, nuts, coffee, and tea.

KOSHER PRACTICES

Kosher means fitting or "proper." Kosher dietary laws (laws of kashrut) concern themselves not only with food, but also with utensils and the conduct of a meal. Here are some of the principles:

Meat and poultry must be obtained from kosher sources, where slaughtering, handling, and processing are supervised.

Meat must come from cloven-hoofed animals that chew their cud. (Leviticus 11:3—*Whatsoever parteth the hoof, and is cloven footed, and cheweth the cud, among the beasts, that shall ye eat.*) There must be no visible traces of blood. Meat must be well done. (Genesis 9:4— *But flesh with the life thereof, which is the blood thereof, shall ye not eat;* and Leviticus 17:10—*I will even set my face against that soul that eateth blood, and will cut him off from among his people.*)

Only fish that have fins and scales may be eaten. Shellfish is not permitted. (Leviticus 11:12—*Whatsoever hath no fins nor scales in the waters, that shall be an abomination unto you.*)

Dairy products and meat may not be eaten at the same meal. (Exodus 23:19—*Thou shalt not seethe a kid in his mother's milk.*) Meat may follow a dairy food, but several hours must elapse after a meat course before a milk product may be eaten. Separate utensils must be used to prepare and serve meat and dairy foods.

Fish, eggs, fruits, vegetables, grains, coffee, tea, and nondairy fats and creamers are neutral (parve) and may be taken at any time.

Passover is a Jewish religious holiday that commemorates the Jews' exodus from Egypt. The observance of Passover requires entirely separate sets of utensils and special dietary observances, particularly the omission and removal of any leavened grain or grain product, such as bread or pasta. (Exodus 13:7—*and there shall no leavened bread be seen with thee, neither shall there be leaven seen with thee in all thy quarters.*)

Kosher commercial products bear symbols that represent certification by different rabbinical organizations. Shown here are two of them.

Six or seven million Americans buy kosher products. Only a fourth of them are Jews who keep kosher homes. Another fourth are Moslems who have similar restrictions with regard to meat. The remainder are Seventh Day Adventists and others who either believe in Jewish dietary laws or think they are getting a "purer" product.

CLEAR LIQUID, LIQUID, AND SOFT DIETS

A clear liquid diet is used when solid or semi-solid foods cannot be tolerated, and when all solid matter must be withheld, even in pureed or liquid suspension form. The following items are allowed: water, apple juice, fat-free broth, bouillon, plain gelatin desserts, fruit ice, tea, and carbonated drinks.

A liquid or full liquid diet is used as a transition between the very restrictive clear liquid diet and a more permissive menu. It also serves people who have difficulty with biting and chewing. In addition to clear liquids, permitted foods include all fruit and vegetable juices, strained cream soups, milk and milk drinks, smooth cooked cereals such as farina, plain yogurt, sherbet, ice cream, smooth pudding, and custard.

A soft diet, sometimes required after surgery or for gastrointestinal or dental problems, adds the following: pureed fruits and vegetables, mashed potatoes, apple sauce, bananas, pureed or finely chopped meat or fowl, cream sauce, gravy, eggs, cottage cheese, butter, margarine, creamy peanut butter, refined white bread, cooked refined cereal, and coffee.

CHAPTER 10

Labels

It is important to read and understand labels. They are well thought out and well designed, and they contain a wealth of information for the consumer.

Ingredients in food products are listed in order of weight. If a frozen dinner is called "Gravy and Turkey" or lists these contents in that order, it means that the product contains more gravy than turkey. If a breakfast cereal names sugar as its first ingredient, it contains more sugar than cereal grain.

Each food label contains a serving size. This has been standardized, so that different manufacturers use comparable quantities. Nevertheless it may be misleading. Spaghetti and other pasta varieties, for example, list nutrition information for two ounce portions. This is not a realistic amount for many spaghetti eaters. Check the serving size; if it is not *your* kind of serving, adjust the nutrition information accordingly.

"Calories" and "Calories from Fat" appear next on the label. If you want to know what *percentage* of the calories comes from fat, multiply *fat* calories by 100 and divide by the calories. Example: tortilla chips, 150 calories, 70 fat calories per serving. Percent of calories from fat: $7000 \div 150 = 47\%$.

"% Daily Value" is the next important entry. Based on a 2000 calorie diet, it heads the list of the important nutrients, and tells us what percent of each nutrient the food product supplies. It shows not only total fat, but also saturated fat; not only carbohydrates, but also fiber and sugar. (It is no longer possible to conceal the total sugar content by separately listing small amounts of corn syrup, malt syrup, honey, sucrose, dextrose etc., as some cereals did.)

Vitamins A and C are the only vitamins regularly listed. Among the minerals, sodium, calcium and iron are required. If a food product is enriched or fortified with any other vitamin or mineral, or if a special claim is made for any one of them, this must then be included on the label.

The FDA examined many health claims before deciding on which ones to permit. Until recently this matter was unregulated, and, as a result, 40 percent of new food products introduced to the marketplace made health claims of one sort or another! As of now, several food–health relationships may be alluded to on the label. These are:

Nutrition Facts

Serving Size 1 cup (228g)
Serving Per Container 2

Amount Per Serving

Calories 260 Calories from Fat 120

	% Daily Value*
Total Fat 13g	20%
Saturated Fat 5g	25%
Cholesterol 30mg	10%
Sodium 660mg	20%
Total Cardohydrate 31g	10%
Dietary Fiber 0g	0%
Sugars 5g	
Protein 5g	

Vitamin A 4%	•	Vitamin C 2%
Calcium 15%	•	Iron 4%

* Percent Daily Values are based on a 2,000 calorie diet. Your daily values may be higher or lower depending on your calorie needs:

	Calories	2,000	2,500
Total Fat	Less than	25g	80g
Sat Fat	Less than	20g	25g
Cholesterol	Less than	300mg	300mg
Sodium	Less than	2,400mg	2,400mg
Total Carbohydrate		300g	375g
Dietary Fiber		25g	30g

Calories per gram:
Fat 9 • Carbohydrate 4 • Protein 4

- Calcium and a reduced risk of osteoporosis
- Low sodium and a reduced risk of high blood pressure
- A diet low in saturated fat and cholesterol and rich in vegetables, fruits and high-grain fiber (especially soluble fiber), and a reduced risk of heart disease
- A diet low in fat and high in fiber-containing grains, fruits and vegetables, and a reduced risk of some types of cancer

These associations may not be stated as facts, but as carefully worded suggestions. Several other medical claims are *not* allowed, among them the claim that fish reduces the risk of cardiovascular disease and the claim that antioxidants reduce cancer risk.

Descriptive terms on food products must *also* follow specific rules.

Calorie free: fewer than 5 calories per serving
Low calorie: 40 calories or less per serving
Reduced or fewer calories: at least 25 percent fewer calories per serving than reference food

Fat free: less than 0.5 gm of fat per serving
Low fat: 3 gm or less per serving
Reduced or less fat: at least 25 percent less per serving than reference food
Saturated fat free: less than 0.5 gm of saturated fat per servings; also trans fatty acids do not exceed 1 percent of total fat
Low saturated fat: 1 gm or less per serving and not more than 15 percent of calories from saturated fatty acids
Reduced or less saturated fat: at least 25 percent less per serving than reference food

Cholesterol free: less than 2 mg of cholesterol and 2 gm or less of saturated fat per serving
Low cholesterol: 20 mg or less, and 2 gm or less of saturated fat per serving
Reduced or less cholesterol: at least 25 percent less, and 2 gm or less of saturated fat per serving than reference food.

Sugar free: less than 0.5 gm of sugar per serving
No added sugar: no sugars added during processing, including ingredients that contain sugar (e.g. fruit juice)
Reduced sugar: at least 25 percent less sugar per serving than reference food

High fiber: 5 gm of fiber, or more, per serving
Good source of fiber: 2.5 gm to 4.9 gm per serving
More or added fiber: at least 2.5 gm more per serving than reference food

Sodium free: less than 5 mg of sodium per serving

Very low sodium: 35 mg or less per serving (No other item can carry a "very low" designation)

Low sodium: 140 mg or less per serving

Reduced or less sodium: at least 25 percent less per serving than reference food

Light or lite: contains one-third fewer calories or half the fat of reference food. Also the sodium in such a food has been reduced 50 percent. "Light" can also describe color or texture, as long as the meaning is made clear

Manufactured packaged foods fall under the jurisdiction of the FDA.

Meat and poultry are supervised by the Food Safety and Inspection Service (FSIS), currently an arm of the U.S. Department of Agriculture, but probably destined to join the FDA or to become an independent agency. At present there is little more than visual inspection of the seven *billion* pieces of poultry sold annually.

Labeling of these foods is on a *voluntary* basis at "point of purchase," usually the food market. The same is true for game, fish, shellfish and produce, overseen by the FDA. Point of purchase information on these food items can be provided by the store in the form of brochures, stickers or posters. The store should also furnish handling and cooking instructions, particularly for ground meat and ground poultry.

The method of informing the public is flexible, but the terms are clearly defined.

Fresh: not a reliable designation at the present time. Poultry that has been stored or shipped at temperatures below 32 degrees may be called fresh; this involves half of all chickens and turkeys in food markets. New legislation would require that such poultry be labeled "previously frozen."

Lean: the food contains less than 10 gm of fat, less than 4 gm of saturated fat, and less than 95 mg of cholesterol per serving and per 100 gm, (about 3½ oz).

Extra lean: the food contains less than 5 gm of fat, less than 2 gm of saturated fat and less than 95 mg of cholesterol per serving and per 100 gm.

Prime, choice, select: terms pertaining to taste qualities, rather than nutritional value or freshness. Prime beef is usually the tastiest and most tender, because it is the most "marbled" (with fat!).

Some foods do not require any labels. Restaurant and airline food, bakery and deli items, foods that contain no nutrients, such as coffee and tea, some very small or odd-shaped packages, and foods produced by small companies are exempt. Incidentally, it has been found that the labeling on national brands is quite accurate; labels on products that are packaged and sold in local areas are much less reliable. A jumbo bran muffin, promoted as "natural" at the deli counter, could supply up to a thousand calories to the unwary snacker.

Substances administered to animals, or added to any food before it is processed by the manufacturer, need not be declared. This includes antibiotics and hormones given to livestock and poultry, and preservatives or irradiation used on ingredients before they went to the processor.

To be called a *"dietary supplement"* a product must provide at least half of the recommended allowances of vitamins and minerals.

The term *"fortified"* means that something not normally found in the food has been added to it; a good example is milk fortified with vitamin D.

The term *"enriched"* means that some ingredient that was lost during processing has been put back; an example is flour, enriched with B vitamins.

"Natural" and "organic" are labels that carry great appeal, but they are not well-defined terms, and can be used and misused to mean many things. Unless clearly defined, and certified, they are not necessarily stamps of good nutritional quality.

Net weight includes everything inside the container: the syrup of canned fruit, the oil in the sardine can, the liquid in a jar of olives.

Dates on food products cannot be understood unless the type of dating is specified. The date may indicate when the product was packed, or the last recommended sell date (which usually allows for a few extra storage days at home), or the expiration date which is the final date on which the food should be considered wholesome, or the freshness date, indicating the last day a product will be fresh-tasting. Some dates are in code and cannot be deciphered by the consumer at all. This is particularly true of canned foods, whose shelf life is long, but certainly not infinite.

Shown below are some abbreviations associated with food labels.

FDA   Food and Drug Administration

FSIS   Food Safety and Inspection Service

DV   Daily Value: a reference value on the label which pertains to the percent of a nutrient that one serving of the food product provides.

RDA   Recommended Daily Dietary Allowance: the estimated daily nutritional requirement, as formulated and published by the National Research Council. Values quoted in this volume apply to healthy nonpregnant adults only. Recommendations for children and pregnant or lactating women should be made by a physician.

RDI   Reference Daily Intake: a reference value *not* shown on the label, used to compute DV. It closely resembles the RDA, but is based on *average* requirements, without regard to age, sex, or special needs

UPC   Universal Product Code. This is the patch of lines and numbers that serves as a code for food and nonfood products, and can be scanned at checkout counters for product identification and price

CHAPTER 11

Calories

As applied to living organisms, calories are a measure of energy: the energy taken in as food, and the energy expended by activities and bodily processes.

Caloric requirements vary greatly, depending on age, size, and activity. A small sedentary elderly woman may need 1,000 calories daily, a large young man doing heavy labor may utilize three or four times that much.

Proteins, carbohydrates, and fats are the three groups of caloric nutrients. Proteins and carbohydrates, in their pure form, provide 4 calories per gram, or 113 calories per ounce. Fats contribute 9 calories per gram, or 255 calories per ounce.

Quantities of Food That Supply About 100 Calories

DAIRY PRODUCTS
Whole milk	5 oz
Skim milk	9 oz
Butter	1 tbs
Cheddar and other hard cheese	1 oz
Low-fat cottage cheese (2%) ½ cup	
Low-fat yogurt	2⅔ cup
Ice cream	1⅓ cup

SPREADS
Oleo	1 tbs
Mayonnaise	1 tbs
Peanut butter	1 tbs

Honey	1½ tbs
Jam	1¾ tbs
MEAT, POULTRY, SEAFOOD (cooked without fat)	
Sirloin steak	1½ oz
Turkey, white meat	2 oz
Cod	3½ oz
Shrimp	10 medium
CEREALS AND CEREAL PRODUCTS	
Oatmeal, cream of wheat or rice	3¾ cup
Wheaties, Cornflakes, Special K	1 cup
Shredded wheat	1¼ biscuits
Spaghetti, cooked	½ cup
VEGETABLES	
Celery	12 stalks
Lettuce, shredded	12 cups
Tomatoes	2 large
Onions, chopped	1½ cups
Green beans, broccoli, cooked	2½ cups
Potato, baked	1 medium
Potatoes, French fried	7 pieces
FRUITS	
Apple	1 medium-large
Banana	1 medium
Cherries	20
Grapefruit	1 large
Grapes	18–30
Orange	1 large
SNACKS	
Potato chips	9 pieces
Saltines	8 pieces
Dry roasted peanuts	2⅔ oz
Jelly beans	15 pieces
Chocolate chip cookies	2 pieces
BEVERAGES	
Orange juice	7 oz
Cola drink	8 oz
Whiskey	1½ oz
Table wine	5 oz
Beer	8 oz

ACTIVITY AND CALORIES

Larger people will spend 100 calories more quickly; smaller people will take longer. In other words, more energy is expended for the same task by a large person than by a small one. The figures given below indicate the approximate number of minutes that it would take a 150-pound individual to work off 100 calories. It takes the expenditure of thirty times that much to achieve a one-pound weight loss!

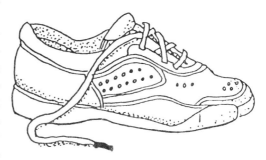

Nevertheless, even though moderate exercise doesn't make up for overeating, a steady regime of exercise does have an effect on weight. Two hundred extra calories expended each day for a year will produce an easy weight loss of twenty pounds.

Time Necessary to Expend 100 Calories

Minutes	Activity
85	Sleeping or resting
77	Reading, watching TV
36	Driving
28	Strolling (3 miles per hour)
26	Tennis, doubles
20	Walking, moderate speed (3½ miles per hour)
19	Social dancing
17	Bicycling, moderate speed
16	Tennis, singles
15	Shoveling snow
10	Jogging
10	Aerobics
9	Swimming
7	Running, 8-minute mile
5	Racing: track, bicycle or swimming

Physical activity is important for the maintenance of good health. The activity may consist of housework, child care, farm labor, or recreational exercise. It should involve several muscle groups, and at times be vigorous enough to raise the pulse rate.

FASCINATING FACTS ABOUT CALORIES

• Calories are all-important in weight loss diets. Fad diets, diet pills, diet books and commercial diet regimes come and go, but it's the calories that count. There are tricks to eating fewer calories (less fat, fewer courses, smaller portions, no seconds, no between-meal snacks), but one method that is *not* recommended is a grossly unbalanced diet. Not only can it cause adverse metabolic effects, but it is unsatisfying, it cannot be maintained over the long haul, and it certainly does not promote good eating habits.

• It pays to be a calorie counter, and not be fooled by popular myth. A cup of creamed cottage cheese has about the same calories as a cup of cooked spaghetti (plain, of course). A cup of low fat fruit yogurt has more calories than a lightly buttered English muffin; it contains almost nine teaspoons of sugar. A glass of orange juice has more calories than the same amount of Coke. An ounce of raisins has more calories than an ounce of jelly beans.

• Substituting 6 ounces of fish for 6 ounces of steak once a week will save over 16,000 calories a year. Switching from a glass of whole milk to skim milk every day will reduce annual calories by more than 23,000. Making sandwiches with turkey breast meat or lean ham instead of bologna or Swiss cheese twice a week results in 17,000 fewer calories. These changes are not only better nutritionally, but, added up, will result in a weight loss of almost 20 pounds over the year.

BODY WEIGHT

Many methods have been devised for determining ideal body weight. For several decades, the Metropolitan Life Insurance tables have been used as a standard. Although useful, they may be flawed in several ways. (1) No allowances are made for age; people normally gain a modest amount of weight as they get older. (2) Great variation is allowed for body types; for example the "desirable" weight of a 5'4" woman can be anything from 114 to 146 pounds. While it is true that some people have larger frames than others, self-assessment is often fallacious. Accurate frame analysis is rarely done by nonprofessionals, and heavy people tend to attribute their overweight to large frames. (3) The tables are based largely on the longevity of policy holders. Since people often lose weight when they are chronically or terminally ill, the statistics may unduly associate low body weight with high mortality. This

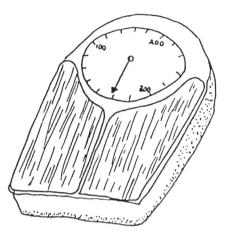

factor would produce a higher ideal weight. (4) Because of the prevalent mix of policy holders at the time that the tables were conceived, the data were based mostly on middle-class white men.

In recent years, tables have been devised that do not differentiate between men and women or body types, but concern themselves only with height and age. Other tables use only height and gender. Some tables aim for extreme leanness. Clearly there is no perfect formula for the perfect weight. Shown below is a table with reasonable criteria. Weight includes a minimum of light clothing (underwear). Height is measured without shoes.

Desirable Weights in Pounds

Height	20–29	30–39	Age 40–49	50–59	60-plus	Avg U.S.
			WOMEN			
4'10	97	102	106	109	111	122
4'11	100	105	109	112	114	
5'	103	108	112	115	117	127
5'1	106	111	115	118	120	
5'2	109	114	118	121	123	132
5'3	112	117	121	124	126	
5'4	115	120	124	127	129	137
5'5	118	123	127	130	132	
5'6	121	126	130	133	135	142
5'7	124	129	133	136	138	
5'8	127	132	136	139	141	147
5'9	130	135	139	142	144	
5'10	133	138	142	145	147	152
			MEN			
5'2	121	125	126	127	126	142
5'3	125	129	130	131	130	
5'4	129	133	134	135	134	154
5'5	133	137	138	139	138	
5'6	137	141	143	144	143	166
5'7	141	145	147	148	147	
5'8	145	149	151	152	151	178
5'9	149	153	155	156	155	
5'10	153	158	160	162	161	190
5'11	157	162	164	165	164	
6'	161	166	168	169	168	202
6'1	166	171	173	174	172	
6'2	171	176	178	179	177	215
6'3	176	181	183	184	181	
6'4	181	186	188	190	187	227

Common Abbreviations, Weights, Measures, Equivalents

Abbreviations

kg = kilogram
gm = gram
mg = milligram
mcg = microgram
L = liter
ml = milliliter
cc = cubic centimeter
lb = pound
oz = ounce
gr = grain
qt = quart
pt = pint
C = cup
fl oz = fluid ounce
tbs = tablespoon
tsp = teaspoon
IU or I.U. = international unit

Equivalents

1 kg = 1000 gm
1 gm = 1000 mg
1 mg = 1000 mcg
1 mcg = 1 millionth gm
1 L = 1000 ml or 1000 cc

1 kg = 2.2 lb
1 lb = 454 gm
1 oz = 28.35 gm
1 gr = 65 mg
1 qt = 2 pt = about 960 ml
1 pt = 2 C = 480 ml
1 C = 8 fl oz = 240 ml
1 fl oz = 30 ml
1 tbs = 15 ml
1 tsp = 5 ml

Index

Entries in bold type indicate the main entry of a topic.